Praise for *100 Questions & Answers About Sports Nutrition and Exercise*

"*100 Questions & Answers About Sports Nutrition and Exercise* is a great addition to any athlete's or coach's library. It provides straightforward explanations for key topics that will help optimize performance. The book's format with easy-to-read tables and *Quick Fact* sections allow readers to immediately access the information they need. Perfect for those pressed for time who need accurate information in one convenient location! Also ideal for nutrition and fitness professionals who need a quick reference guide for commonly asked questions."

Kelli J. Kidd, MS, RD, CSSD
United States Military Academy Sports
Dietitian and Iron-Man Triathlete

"Sports nutrition plays such a vital role in an athlete's performance and overall health, yet, this area is often overlooked by even the most well-intentioned athletes. *100 Questions & Answers About Sports Nutrition and Exercise* is an excellent resource for the entire spectrum of athletes, as it highlights the importance and relevance of nutrition by covering an array of topics that appeal to everyone from novice to professional. The practical information presented is compressive, detailed, and well organized, and allows for immediate application to enhance performance and promote well-being."

Nina M. Schroder, MSW, LCSW-C
Former NCAA Division I Athlete

"Pop culture continues to affect so many areas of our lives. Fitness and diet are no exception. This book is a much needed reference to anyone serious about the 'truth' in exercise programming and nutrition for performance. The authors have done an outstanding job of identifying practical areas that most people are concerned about.

They have presented the responses to those areas in a concise and effective manner. This text will be an outstanding reference for the novice developing a program for themselves or the expert looking for additional means to assist them in explaining the 'truth' about nutrition and exercise planning."

Al Bransdorfer, PhD
U.S. Navy Aerospace Physiologist

100 Questions & Answers About Sports Nutrition and Exercise

Lilah Al-Masri, MS, RD, CSSD, LD
Quest Sports Science Center
Annapolis, MD

Simon Bartlett, PhD, CSCS, ATC
Quest Sports Science Center
Annapolis, MD

JONES AND BARTLETT PUBLISHERS
Sudbury, Massachusetts
BOSTON   TORONTO   LONDON   SINGAPORE

World Headquarters

Jones and Bartlett Publishers	Jones and Bartlett Publishers	Jones and Bartlett Publishers
40 Tall Pine Drive	Canada	International
Sudbury, MA 01776	6339 Ormindale Way	Barb House, Barb Mews
978-443-5000	Mississauga, Ontario L5V 1J2	London W6 7PA
info@jbpub.com	Canada	United Kingdom
www.jbpub.com		

Jones and Bartlett's books and products are available through most bookstores and online booksellers. To contact Jones and Bartlett Publishers directly, call 800-832-0034, fax 978-443-8000, or visit our website, www.jbpub.com.

Substantial discounts on bulk quantities of Jones and Bartlett's publications are available to corporations, professional associations, and other qualified organizations. For details and specific discount information, contact the special sales department at Jones and Bartlett via the above contact information or send an email to specialsales@jbpub.com.

The authors, editor, and publisher have made every effort to provide accurate information. However, they are not responsible for errors, omissions, or for any outcomes related to the use of the contents of this book and take no responsibility for the use of the products and procedures described. Treatments and side effects described in this book may not be applicable to all people; likewise, some people may require a dose or experience a side effect that is not described herein. Drugs and medical devices are discussed that may have limited availability controlled by the Food and Drug Administration (FDA) for use only in a research study or clinical trial. Research, clinical practice, and government regulations often change the accepted standard in this field. When consideration is being given to use of any drug in the clinical setting, the healthcare provider or reader is responsible for determining FDA status of the drug, reading the package insert, and reviewing prescribing information for the most up-to-date recommendations on dose, precautions, and contraindications, and determining the appropriate usage for the product. This is especially important in the case of drugs that are new or seldom used.

Production Credits
Acquisitions Editor: Shoshanna Goldberg
Senior Associate Editor: Amy Bloom
Senior Editorial Assistant: Kyle Hoover
Production Director: Amy Rose
Production Manager: Julie Bolduc
Associate Production Editor: Jessica deMartin
Associate Marketing Manager: Jody Sullivan
V.P., Manufacturing and Inventory Control:
   Therese Connell
Composition: Glyph International
Printing and Binding: Malloy, Inc.

Cover Credits
Cover Design: Carolyn Downer
Cover Printing: Malloy, Inc.
Cover Images: Top left: © Noam
   Armonn/ShutterStock, Inc.; Bottom left:
   © Radin Myroslav/ShutterStock, Inc.; Top
   right: © Shawn Pecor/ShutterStock, Inc.;
   Bottom right: © Photos.com

Library of Congress Cataloging-in-Publication Data
Masri, Lilah Al.
  100 questions & answers about sports nutrition and exercise/Lilah Al Masri, Simon Bartlett.
    p. cm.
  Includes index.
  ISBN 978-0-7637-7886-6 (alk. paper)
  1. Athletes—Nutrition—Miscellanea. 2. Physical fitness—Nutritional
aspects—Miscellanea. 3. Sports. I. Bartlett, Simon. II. Title. III.
Title: 100 questions and answers about sports nutrition and exercise. IV.
Title: One hundred question & answers about sports nutriiton and exercise.
  TX361.A8M374 2011
  613.2'024796—dc22
                              2009052696

6048

Printed in the United States of America
14 13 12 11 10   10 9 8 7 6 5 4 3 2 1

This book is dedicated to all of our family and friends for their encouragement and support.

Contents

Questions 1–15 discuss general sports nutrition, including the following:
- Why should an athlete develop a nutrition and exercise plan?
- What is hunger?
- What should my training plate look like?

Questions 16–34 review general exercise concepts:
- What are the health benefits of regular exercise?
- What are the basic principles of exercise that are needed to optimize training and performance?
- Why should athletes warm up before and cool down after exercise?

Questions 35–48 discuss the timing of meals and snacks:
- What should I eat before exercise?
- Should I eat before an early-morning workout?
- What types of foods should the athlete consume during exercise?

Questions 49–53 discuss vitamins and minerals:
- What role do vitamins play in an athlete's diet?
- What role do minerals play in an athlete's diet?
- What role does calcium play in athletic performance?

Contents

Athletes, coaches, fitness trainers, and the general public are continually striving to achieve a higher level of fitness. As we plan our training and give thought to our nutritional habits, we have a variety of questions. We look for information that is concise and comprehendible to assist us in achieving our goals.

Lilah Al-Masri and Simon Bartlett, who have devoted their lives to the pursuit of excellence in fitness, created *100 Questions & Answers About Sports Nutrition and Exercise* for this purpose. This book provides an excellent source of knowledge, covering an array of exercise and nutritional information for everyone to use in his or her quest to become healthier and more physically fit.

Stephen M. Cooksey
Head Track & Field Coach
U.S. Naval Academy

Sports nutrition and exercise are very popular topics today. Too frequently, athletes are exposed to nutrition and exercise information that is not necessarily accurate or legitimate. Athletes are competitive by nature, and with that competitiveness, they can fall prey to bad advice. Our goal in this book is to present scientifically based, usable, and concrete concepts that provide recreational and elite athletes of all ages with information that will allow them to excel in their respective sports. In addition, this book is designed to debunk the many myths, superstitions, and misinformation that saturate the fields of sports nutrition and exercise. The information in this book is a supplement and is *not* a replacement for an individual nutrition and exercise program that is designed by a sports dietitian and an exercise physiologist, respectively.

The questions and answers in this book were inspired by the most frequent concerns that we have encountered from athletes throughout the years. All of the case studies in this book are based on actual situations and events; therefore, the reader can be confident that the recommendations provide real-world solutions that work when implemented correctly. Our intentions are to take out the guesswork and replace it with simple and easy-to-use strategies.

We acknowledge all of the athletes who we have had the privilege of encountering over the years. If it were not for their curiosity, we would never have been inspired to write this invaluable book.

Lilah Al-Masri and Simon Bartlett have teamed up to combine their expertise in sports nutrition and exercise physiology with Olympic, collegiate, and professional athletes to create this book. Both have considerable experience with developing nutrition and exercise programs for athletes in a variety of sports. Working with trainers, coaches, dietitians, physicians, and parents has helped to expand their expertise to develop this book and fill a niche that was missing. As nutrition and exercise researchers and consultants, Al-Masri and Bartlett have coached clients to achieve successful outcomes in a variety of athletic endeavors. This book completes your understanding of nutrition and exercise interactions by concisely answering your questions while providing individualized help with understandable examples and illustrations based on real-world experience. I am certain you'll enjoy this book and use it as a reference because of the sound advice and recommendations for athletes desiring to meet their goals with nutrition and exercise.

Laura Nihan, PhD, MS Ed, RD
Retired LTC USAF, Registered Dietitian

General Sports Nutrition

Why should an athlete develop a nutrition and exercise plan?

What is hunger?

What should my training plate look like?

More . . .

Athletes must have a basic foundation in both general and sports nutrition to benefit fully from its implementation. Athletes who fail to learn and implement the basics of nutrition will be at a distinct disadvantage when it comes to training, competing, and recovering. Part One familiarizes the athlete with common questions and answers that will benefit all athletes who are serious about improving their performance.

1. Why should an athlete develop a nutritional and exercise plan?

Athletes need to feed their bodies continually in order to perform at their peak. Practice, game, and tournament play place specific nutritional and physical demands on the athlete. These demands can be met with a well-designed nutrition and exercise program. Achieving peak performance requires that athletes understand and implement the fundamental principles of sports nutrition and exercise science for their sport. Key strategies for a successful performance will include preparation before, during, and after exercise. For athletes to achieve optimal performance, they must take into account the physical demands of their sport (intensity, duration, frequency), their size, and the environment (temperature, humidity, etc.) in which they practice and compete. All of these factors contribute to the sport-specific nutritional and exercise plan that will assist the athletes in achieving their athletic goals.

2. What is hunger?

Hunger is an unpleasant sensation that an individual experiences when circulating **blood glucose** levels decrease; it can be alleviated through eating. Hunger should be avoided by all athletes to help prevent energy loss. Athletes must be aware of the signs of hunger.

Key strategies for a successful performance will include preparation before, during, and after exercise.

Hunger

An unpleasant sensation that an individual experiences when circulating blood glucose decreases; it can be alleviated through eating.

Blood glucose

Amount of glucose circulating in the bloodstream.

Hunger appears in various ways, but most athletes recognize hunger by only **stomach pangs**. After stomach pangs have been sensed, too many hours have passed without feeding the body. Other hunger cues can include **fatigue**, poor concentration, headaches, irritability, shakiness, and sleep disturbances. These symptoms are usually felt before the stomach pangs and should be acted on immediately to prevent more intense hunger and additional energy loss. Being able to detect your body's hunger cues is important, as this will stabilize energy and metabolism throughout the day, leading to superior mental and physical performance.

Stomach pangs
A sharp feeling of pain in the stomach.

Fatigue
Physical or mental exhaustion from overexertion.

■ *Case Study*

Nadia, a 20-year-old collegiate softball pitcher, presents to the sports dietitian with complaints of headaches and fatigue. She is confused about why she continues to get headaches, as she drinks plenty of water throughout the day and during practices. Nadia practices twice a day: 60 to 90 minutes of conditioning in the morning and 2 to 3 hours of skills practice in the afternoon. Nadia was asked to keep a 1-week food and exercise log that also emphasized rating her hunger level throughout the day. On review, the sports dietitian noted that Nadia had a hard time judging her hunger level, causing her to skip meals and snacks. Nadia rarely feels hungry throughout the day, but she often gets a headache a few hours after her morning practice and when she is studying in the evening. The sports dietitian reviewed some of the common signs of hunger with Nadia. Nadia was surprised that hunger cues also include fatigue, poor concentration, headaches, irritability, shakiness, and sleep disturbances—not just stomach pangs. Nadia recognized that she often experiences one or more of these symptoms throughout the day. Nadia, together with the sports

General Sports Nutrition

dietitian, developed a consistent meal and snack plan that would fit around her busy academic and athletic schedule. After just one day of following the plan, Nadia reported that her headaches subsided and her concentration in the classroom and on the field had greatly improved.

3. What should my training plate look like?

Carbohydrates

The main source of energy for all body functions, particularly brain and muscle functions; necessary for the metabolism of other nutrients.

Protein

Made up of amino acids that act as the building blocks for muscles, blood, skin, hair, nails, and the internal organs.

Fat

A wide group of compounds that may be either solid or liquid at room temperature.

Complex carbohydrates

A carbohydrate composed of two or more linked simple-sugar molecules.

Lean proteins

Protein sources that are low in saturated or trans fats, including beans, nuts, nut butters, eggs, chicken, turkey, fish, and soy.

An athlete's plate should be balanced between **carbohydrate**, **protein**, and **fat** food sources. Choose **complex carbohydrates**, **lean proteins**, unsaturated fats, and plenty of fruits and vegetables to ensure variety in the diet. The following total calorie intake is recommended: carbohydrates, 50% to 60%; proteins, 15% to 20%; and fats, 20% to 30%. Carbohydrates include fruits, vegetables, breads, rice, pasta, potatoes, cereal, oatmeal, pretzels, and crackers. Lean proteins include chicken and turkey without the skin, fish, lean cuts of beef and pork, eggs, beans, nuts, nut butters, soy, and low-fat dairy products (skim and 1%). Healthy fats include oils, nuts, seeds, fatty fish, avocado, and nut butters. **Figure 1** represents what an athlete's training plate should look like in relationship to the distribution of carbohydrates, proteins, and fats. A specific designation for fats is not included on the plate diagram, as fats are sprinkled in throughout the day in the foods that are consumed and in the way foods are prepared (sautéing, stir frying, and using oil-based dressings). Athletes can easily use the figure as a visual guide for proper eating both at home and on the road.

Quick Fact

Add a variety of colors to your plate; eating an assortment of fruits and vegetables will provide nutrients and flavor to your meals.

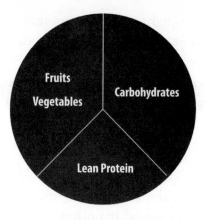

Figure 1   An Athlete's Training Plate.

4. Why are carbohydrates important for exercise?

Carbohydrates are the single most important source of energy for athletic performance. They are a rapid source of fuel to the working muscle and are burned efficiently with or without the presence of oxygen. Carbohydrates are **oxidized** (broken down) three times faster than fat and are the predominant energy source for fueling both **aerobic** and **anaerobic** activity.

Carbohydrates are stored in the body's muscle cells as **glycogen** and can provide the athlete with approximately 2,000 to 2,400 calories of energy. Eating sufficient amounts of carbohydrate in the daily diet (more than 50%) will help the body preserve its muscle protein and assist in the use of fat as a fuel. Consuming low-carbohydrate diets is not recommended, as they cause a decrease in muscle glycogen stores. This glycogen decrease can lead to premature muscle fatigue during exercise and may result in the body using its muscle protein as a source of energy. Athletes who

Oxidized

A chemical reaction with oxygen.

Aerobic

In the presence of air or oxygen.

Anaerobic

In the absence of air or oxygen.

Glycogen

The major carbohydrate stored in animal cells, mainly in the muscle cells and some in the liver. Glycogen is converted to glucose and released into circulation, as needed, by the body.

General Sports Nutrition

need to lose weight will discover that carbohydrates aid in the fat-burning process, as fat burns in a carbohydrate flame.

Nerve conduction

The transmission of impulses throughout the nerves in the body.

Carbohydrates should make up 50% or more of an athlete's daily food intake; anything less than 50% can compromise muscle strength, muscle endurance, power, mental focus, and recovery.

Carbohydrate loading

A method of increasing a cell's glycogen content beyond its usual capacity.

Quick Fact

Very high-carbohydrate diets can raise blood triglyceride levels, leading to increased fat stores and weight gain.

Carbohydrates are the key to muscle contraction, **nerve conduction**, and brain function. Carbohydrates should make up 50% or more of an athlete's daily food intake; anything less than 50% can compromise muscle strength, muscle endurance, power, mental focus, and recovery. Carbohydrates are essential before, during, and after exercise in order for the athlete to attain optimal performance and recovery.

The average athlete has the capacity to store approximately 400 to 500 grams of carbohydrate as glycogen in the body. Glycogen is stored in the body at three sites: muscle cells, liver, and blood (**Figure 2**). Muscle cells are the largest source, storing approximately 300 to 400 grams (1,200 to 1,400 kcal). The liver is the second largest storage site, containing approximately 75 to 100 grams (300 to 400 kcal). Blood is the smallest site, circulating approximately 25 grams (100 kcal). Training and **carbohydrate loading** positively influence the amount of muscle glycogen stored.

The glycogen that is used during exercise is specific to the muscle being used. Although there are 300 to 400 grams of total glycogen stored throughout the muscles, only a certain percentage can be used, depending on which muscles are activated. A runner, for example, will use the glycogen stores in the muscles of the lower extremities (hamstrings, calves, and quadriceps), whereas

General Sports Nutrition

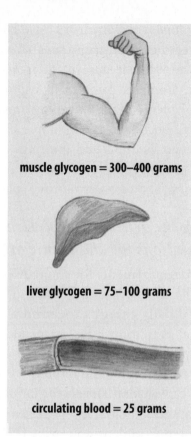

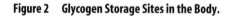

Figure 2   Glycogen Storage Sites in the Body.

the glycogen in the upper extremity muscles (biceps, triceps, shoulders, and back) will be used only marginally.

5. What are the differences between simple and complex carbohydrates?

Carbohydrates are either simple or complex. **Simple carbohydrates** raise blood sugar levels quickly. Examples include bananas, raisins, white breads, and energy gels. After simple carbohydrates have been digested, they enter the bloodstream as **glucose** to provide a rapid source of energy to the brain and exercising muscles. Conversely, **complex carbohydrates** raise blood sugar levels more slowly. Examples include whole-grain cereals, oatmeal, whole-grain breads, beans, and apples with

Simple carbohydrates

A form of carbohydrate that exists as a monosaccharide or disaccharide.

Glucose

One of the most commonly occurring simple sugars in nature. Humans rely on glucose for cellular energy.

Complex carbohydrates

a carbohydrate composed of two or more linked simple-sugar molecules.

skin. After complex carbohydrates have been digested, they will enter the bloodstream at a slower rate than simple carbohydrates because of their higher **dietary fiber** content. Complex carbohydrates provide a long-term source of energy to the exercising muscle and have a higher nutritional value than simple carbohydrates, providing certain vitamins and minerals. Each type of carbohydrate plays a specific role in the athlete's training, competition, and recovery nutrition plan.

6. What are the general carbohydrate recommendations for endurance athletes?

Carbohydrate requirements for endurance athletes will depend on the intensity and duration of the exercise or sport, **total daily energy expenditure**, gender, and environmental conditions. Recommended guidelines for carbohydrate intake range between 5 and 12 grams of carbohydrates per kilogram of body weight. **Table 1** depicts daily carbohydrate needs for various endurance exercise durations. Total body glycogen content can last an endurance athlete approximately 90 to 120 minutes of continuous endurance exercise. Athletes engaged in high-intensity, short-duration activities such as sprinting and strength training have a unique carbohydrate requirement. These types of activities can

Dietary fiber

A complex carbohydrate obtained from plant sources. It is not digestible by humans. Although dietary fiber provides no energy for cellular activity, it does help maintain a healthy digestive system, lower blood cholesterol levels, and regulate blood glucose levels.

Total daily energy expenditure

Total amount of calories (energy) expended by the body over a 24-hour period.

Table 1   Recommended Carbohydrate Requirements for Various Endurance Activities

Duration of Exercise	Carbohydrate Recommendations
1 hour of exercise per day	5 to 7 grams of carbohydrate per kilogram
Endurance: 1 to 3 hours of exercise per day	7 to 10 grams of carbohydrate per kilogram
Ultra endurance: 3 to 5 hours of exercise per day	10 to 12 grams of carbohydrate per kilogram

reach an intensity of 90% to 100% of maximal effort and can drain glycogen stores in less than 45 minutes.

7. What is the role of protein in the body?

Protein is a crucial nutrient that is required for growth and repair of muscle and other body tissues. Additionally, protein plays a large role in the formation of **hormones**, hemoglobin (blood), **enzymes**, and **antibodies**. Proteins are comprised of **amino acids**, and unlike carbohydrates, they are not stored in the muscles cells as a source of energy. The **recommended dietary intake** for protein should range between 15% and 20% of an athlete's overall diet. Most athletes usually get this amount of protein from their daily food intake. Overconsumption of protein may lead to increased fat storage and dehydration, and long-term use may cause kidney damage. Good sources of lean proteins include nuts/nut butters, eggs, beans, chicken, turkey, low-fat dairy products, soy, and fish.

8. What are the general protein requirements for athletes?

Protein requirements for athletes are variable and depend on the intensity and duration of the exercise or sport, total daily energy expenditure, and gender. Protein needs can be adequately met through diet as long as **total energy intake** is sufficient. Boosting protein intake above the recommended amounts will not provide an additional benefit to the athlete because there is a limit to the rate at which lean muscle mass can accrue. The overconsumption of protein, in excess of 2 grams per kilogram of body weight per day, could potentially lead to acute as well as chronic kidney damage. Athletes with kidney disease should be aware of the dangers of consuming high-protein diets. Daily protein requirements for endurance and strength athletes are listed in **Table 2**.

Hormone

A complex chemical substance produced in one part or organ of the body that initiates or regulates the activity of an organ or group of cells in another part.

Enzymes

Proteins that accelerate chemical reactions.

Antibodies

Part of the immune system that helps to combat and neutralize foreign bodies such as viruses, bacteria, and parasites.

Amino acids

The basic structural building units of proteins.

Recommended dietary intake

The daily amount of nutrients needed to satisfy approximately 98% of healthy individuals.

Total energy intake

Total amount of calories (energy) needed by the body over a 24-hour period.

General Sports Nutrition

Table 2   Recommended Protein Requirements for Various Types of Exercise

Type of Exercise	Protein Recommendations
1 hour of exercise per day	0.8 grams of protein per kilogram
Endurance athlete, 1 to 3 hours of exercise per day	1.2 to 1.4 grams of protein per kilogram
Strength athlete	1.6 to 1.7 grams of protein per kilogram

9. What are the potential health consequences of consuming more than the recommended amount of protein in the diet?

Athletes should be aware of the potential health consequences associated with consuming higher than recommended amounts of dietary protein. High dietary protein intake can lead to numerous health consequences (**Table 3**).

Table 3   Possible Health Consequences of the Overconsumption of Protein

Consequence	Explanation
Low energy	Overconsumption of protein may cause a decrease in carbohydrate consumption
Dehydration	More water is needed to break down and rid the body of protein **metabolites**
Weight loss	Proteins have a higher **satiety** value
Decreased total calorie intake	Early satiety causes decreased overall calorie consumption
Vitamin inadequacies	Proteins do not provide all key vitamins and minerals
Potential bone **decalcification**	Interferes with calcium absorption
Decreased liver and kidney function	High-protein diets may strain the kidneys and liver by making them work harder to rid the body of protein metabolites
Possible increase in fat mass	Overconsumption of protein can be converted and stored as fat

Metabolites

A substance produced by the process of metabolism or vital for a certain metabolic process.

Satiety

Being full or satisfied.

Decalcification

A loss of calcium from teeth and bones.

10. Why is fat an essential part of an athlete's diet?

Fat can be an important source of long-term energy during exercise. It protects and insulates body organs and is necessary for absorption of **fat-soluble vitamins** (A, D, E, and K). Recommended fat intake is 20% to 30% of an athlete's daily food intake. If an athlete consumes a diet that is too low in fat (less than 15%), his or her health may be adversely affected. The side effects of a low-fat diet include dry skin, brittle nails, hair loss, decreased protection of organs, and a fat-soluble vitamin deficiency that leads to poor physical and mental performance.

11. What are the two principle types of fat?

The two principle types of fat in the diet are saturated and unsaturated. **Saturated fat** and **trans fat** are often referred to as the "bad" fat and can lead to high cholesterol, heart disease, weight gain, and poor mental and physical performance. Saturated fats are found in foods such as candy, baked goods, ice cream, whole and 2% milk products, cheese, red meats, and fried foods. Saturated fat should be consumed in moderation, ideally less than 10% of total fat intake. **Unsaturated fats**, including **polyunsaturated fats** and **monounsaturated fats**, are often referred to as the "good" fats, as they are essential to health and may protect against heart disease. Unsaturated fats are found in liquid oils (olive oil, canola oil, and peanut oil), nuts, seeds, avocados, and fish. Eating a diet that is low in saturated fats and higher in unsaturated fats can have a positive impact on the athlete's health and sports performance.

Fat-soluble vitamins

A group of vitamins that do not dissolve easily in water and require dietary fat for intestinal absorption and transport into the bloodstream. The fat-soluble vitamins are A, D, E, and K.

If an athlete consumes a diet that is too low in fat (less than 15%), his or her health may be adversely affected.

Saturated fat

Fat that can cause an increase in cholesterol levels and that increases the risk for heart disease.

Trans fat

Considered to be an unhealthy source of fat that often leads to cardiovascular disease if ingested in high amounts.

Unsaturated fat

A heart-healthy fat that has the potential to lower cholesterol levels and reduce heart disease.

General Sports Nutrition

Polyunsaturated fat

A type of unsaturated fat that has been shown to prevent heart disease.

Monounsaturated fat

A type of fat that is shown to reduce the incidences of heart disease.

Bonking

A condition in which an athlete experiences extreme fatigue and an inability to maintain the current level of activity. It is also known as "hitting the wall" and results when the body has depleted muscle and liver glycogen levels.

12. Should my nutritional strategies differ before competition versus practice? What should I eat if I have only less than 2 hours between games?

The strategies that an athlete has developed for practice should remain consistent in the competitive arena. The athlete must remain well fueled with high-carbohydrate foods and fluids during competition to help prevent **bonking**, gastrointestinal upset, cramping, and excessive muscle tissue damage. During tournament play, when there are usually multiple events in 1 day and often little time between events to eat full meals, frequent snacking will be essential to the athlete's performance. Refueling is important to restore severely depleted glycogen stores as quickly as possible in order to perform effectively during the next game.

■ *Case Study*

Natalina is a 21-year-old varsity soccer midfielder. Her position requires a lot of endurance and sprinting during the 90-minute game. In the championship tournament, she will play two games per day with less than 2 hours between each game. She must consume foods that taste good, provide the necessary energy to fuel her performance for the second match, and are quickly digestable so that they do not bother her stomach. Natalina should consume a snack that is high in carbohydrates and low in proteins and fats immediately after the first game. Some excellent snacks include a bagel with jam and a sports drink, a piece of fruit and/or a granola bar and sports drink, or graham crackers and low-fat chocolate milk. These foods will be digested and enter the circulation quickly, helping Natalina to recover some of her energy stores in time for the next game and thus maintain a higher level of performance.

A word of caution: Natalina should avoid consuming solids foods within 30 minutes of her second game. This will allow enough time for proper digestion and help to prevent stomach upset. During the 30 minutes before the game, Natalina should consume approximately 8 to 16 ounces (1 to 2 cups) of water or sports drinks to ensure adequate hydration.

Rob's (women's collegiate swim coach) comments:

Being a coach of a women's swim team, I have observed many different ways that the athletes approach their nutritional strategies during practices and meets. Sadly, these are not always conducive to optimal performance. Many do not think about what to consume; rather, they consume whatever is available to them at the time. As a coach, I know that my athletes cannot get stronger or faster without choosing the proper foods; therefore, I strongly encourage my athletes to consult with the sports dietitian to educate them in helping to make proper food choices at home and on the road that will enhance their performance and recovery.

13. When should an athlete introduce new sports drinks and/or foods?

A variety of foods/beverages are on the market for athletes to consume. These products vary in caloric content, taste, texture, size, and nutrient content. No single product satisfies every athlete's nutritional needs. It is important for an athlete to experiment with various products during practice and *not* during competition. An athlete should not try new foods, energy bars, energy gels, or sports drinks for the first time before or during a major competition or event, as this may result in gastrointestinal problems, causing impaired athletic performance.

14. What are the common causes of gastrointestinal distress in athletes?

Gastrointestinal distress

Distress that occurs in the upper or lower gastrointestinal tracts that can negatively impact sports performance.

Gastrointestinal distress is unfortunately common in many athletes. Symptoms in the upper and lower part of the gastrointestinal tract can negatively impact performance during exercise and may also be felt after exercise. Symptoms in the upper gastrointestinal tract include heartburn, burping, nausea, and/or vomiting. Symptoms in the lower gastrointestinal tract include cramping, bloating, gas, diarrhea, constipation, and/or gastrointestinal bleeding. Several factors can contribute to gastrointestinal distress in athletes, some of which are in the athlete's control and others that are not. These factors are mode of activity (sport), intensity of exercise, age, gender, anxiety level, hydration status, beverage consumption, fiber intake, overconsumption of "sports" foods, medications, supplements, and timing of meals, snacks, and fluids.

1. Sport: The type of activity or sport the athlete is training and competing in may affect gastrointestinal symptoms. Sports that involve jostling (or up and down movements) during activity tend to cause more gastrointestinal distress than those that are more stable. For instance, athletes who participate in running and triathlon events or teams sports such as soccer, basketball, or lacrosse may experience more gastrointestinal distress than athletes who participate in swimming, cycling, or water polo.

2. Intensity: Exercise intensity can influence gastrointestinal symptoms. The more intense the exercise (such as sprinting), the slower are the digestion and absorption rate from the stomach, leading to potential gastrointestinal problems.

3. Age: Experience can be a factor that influences gastrointestinal symptoms. Older adults often pay more

attention to what foods and fluids they are consuming and how these products can positively or negatively affect their performance. Younger athletes tend to consume foods that they enjoy without thinking about the consequences that these foods will have during exercise. Age may not always be a positive, however. As athletes age, gastrointestinal motility may slow, resulting in decreased rates of digestion, absorption, and excretion, leading to an increased incidence of gastrointestinal upset.

4. Gender: Women more often complain of gastrointestinal distress since females have a slower gastric-emptying rate than men (influenced by estrogen). Hormone increases during the menstrual cycle tend to increase the symptoms of lower gastrointestinal distress (cramping, bloating, gas, diarrhea, constipation, and/or gastrointestinal bleeding). Menstrual cramping has also been associated with diarrhea. Experienced female athletes are generally more aware of their body's response to hormonal fluctuations than younger, less experienced athletes.

5. Anxiety: Athletes who tend to experience high anxiety levels before training and/or competition often experience gastrointestinal problems because of decreased gut motility and suppressed hunger. Highly anxious athletes who consume foods or fluids before exercise are generally the most susceptible to gastrointestinal distress. These athletes may feel nauseated and vomit before an event and generally avoid pre-workout meals and snacks. Ironically, avoiding a pre-race or pre-game meal or snack can also cause gastrointestinal problems in addition to promoting early-onset fatigue. Athletes should experiment with various types and amounts of foods and fluids to see what works best for them (see Question 35).

6. Hydration status: The athlete's sweat rate determines the optimal amount of fluid needed during exercise (see Question 41). There is a physiological limit to the amount of fluid that can be emptied from the stomach into the small intestine and eventually into the circulation. If the athlete consumes more fluid than can be digested, the athlete will likely experience an uncomfortable "sloshing" feeling in the stomach, which can cause vomiting and/or cramping. The amount of fluid tolerated in the stomach will depend on the dynamics of the sport and the individual athlete. Athletes should experiment with various types and amounts of foods and fluids to see what works best for them (see Question 13).

7. Beverage consumption: Consuming beverages that contain caffeine, alcohol, and carbonation or are greater than 8% carbohydrate concentration can significantly alter gastric-emptying rates. Higher concentrations of carbohydrate and carbonation in a beverage generally slow stomach emptying, which can cause a strong sensation of fullness and decreased consumption of fluids that may adversely affect the athlete's hydration status.

8. Fiber intake: Diets that are too high or too low in fiber may delay or speed up gastric-emptying rates. Diets that are higher in fiber content will delay gastric emptying, whereas diets low in fiber can accelerate gastric emptying. Athletes should keep fibrous foods to a minimum before exercise or competitions to prevent potential gastrointestinal problems.

9. Overconsumption of "sports" foods: Consuming too many foods that have a high carbohydrate and/or high protein and high fat content in a short period before exercise may cause gastrointestinal distress. Athletes should read labels carefully before

consuming sports food or fluids to ensure that they do not overconsume a particular nutrient.

10. Medications: Excessive use of over-the-counter nonsteroidal anti-inflammatory pain medications, such as ibuprofen, Aleve, and Motrin, may have side effects such as irritation of the stomach lining. This stomach irritation, if severe, may lead to ulcers or other serious complications. An athlete who is suffering from an acute or chronic injury should consult with a healthcare provider on the appropriate use of over-the-counter medications.

11. Supplements: Some supplements are known to react with the stomach, whereas others may contain certain products that the athlete may not be able to tolerate. For example, iron supplements may cause constipation and nausea if taken on an empty stomach. Athletes should consult with a **registered dietitian** regarding any questions or concerns that they may have about supplement use and implications.

12. Timing of meals, snacks, and fluids: Consuming meals, snacks, or fluids too close to the start of exercise or consuming products that may not optimize gastric emptying can have negative outcomes for the athlete. For example, consuming a large amount of dried fruits, fresh fruits, and beans or a high intake of fruit juices before a workout may lead to bloating, gas, and/or diarrhea.

Gastrointestinal distress is likely the result of poor timing or inadequate knowledge or experience. Athletes must educate themselves on the potential causes of gastrointestinal distress and must listen to their bodies. Athletes may want to experiment with various foods and fluids during practice to establish a plan that reduces gastrointestinal issues. Understand that not all

Registered dietitian

An individual trained to provide food and nutrition information and who has successfully passed the national registration exam for registered dietitians.

Gastrointestinal distress is likely the result of poor timing or inadequate knowledge or experience.

gastrointestinal issues are preventable, but with the help of a sports dietitian, the instances can be substantially reduced.

15. Why is sleep important, and how much do I need?

Sleep is essential to life and is as vital to the body as food and oxygen. One of the most common concerns of athletes is sleep. How much should athletes get, and what happens when they are unable to fulfill their sleep requirement?

Sleep requirements for maintaining optimal health as well as physical and mental performance is 8.0 to 8.5 hours a night; however, some people require more or less. Approximately 70% of adult Americans are getting less than 8 hours of sleep per night, which means that most people, including athletes, are somewhat sleep deprived. An athlete who requires 8 hours of sleep per night and is only getting 7 hours will, by the end of the week, accrue 7 hours of sleep debt. A sleep debt of this magnitude is equivalent to the loss of one full night of sleep. Some of the common reasons for sleep deprivation in athletes include stress, workload, training early in the morning or late at night, overtraining, or medical conditions, as well as alcohol and stimulant consumption.

Sleep debt is cumulative and must be restored as soon as possible. If the debt is not repaid, it will roll over to the following week. Athletes will then find themselves experiencing excessive sleepiness during the day and will likely fall asleep at inappropriate times and places, such as behind the wheel of the car, at work, or in the classroom. The first 48 hours of total sleep deprivation has been shown to have deleterious effects on mental capacity only. Physical effects will not manifest until 72 hours.

The body will find a way to catch up, and the longer the sleep debt goes on, the harder it will be to stay awake and perform. Another consequence of sleep deprivation is overeating. Research has shown that those who do not get enough sleep or have a hard time staying asleep will crave higher calorie foods and tend to overeat the next day. Studies have also shown that individuals who suffer from chronic sleep deprivation experience higher incidences of heart disease, obesity, diabetes, and ulcers.

There are two stages to the sleep cycle: the first stage is **non-rapid eye movement** (NREM), and the second stage is **rapid eye movement** (REM). After falling asleep, an individual will enter NREM sleep first where very little dreaming occurs. The purpose behind NREM sleep is to help the body physically repair itself from the previous day's activities. REM sleep, on the other hand, involves a substantial amount of dreaming and is essential to helping the individual recover mentally. During the REM cycle, the mind attempts to process and organize all of the information that it has encountered during the day. The REM cycle is a very active portion of sleep, even though the individual is unable to move; this is analogous to an automobile with the accelerator pressed down and the brake on at the same time. Both the NREM and REM stages are critical to physical and mental reparation. Alcohol consumption and certain medications have been demonstrated to disrupt the REM cycle and should be avoided before bedtime.

The following conditions are necessary to induce healthy sleep:

1. Keep the room dark. If light is able to penetrate into a room, it may interfere with a person's ability to fall and stay asleep; keep the room as dark as possible by using blackout curtains and/or a sleep mask.

General Sports Nutrition

Non-rapid eye movement (NREM)

The first stage of sleep where very little dreaming occurs. The purpose behind non-rapid eye movement sleep is to help the body physically repair itself from the previous day's activities.

Rapid eye movement (REM)

This second stage of sleep involves a substantial amount of dreaming and is essential to helping individuals recover mentally. During the rapid eye movement cycle, the mind attempts to process and organize all of the information that it has encountered during the day.

2. The room should be quiet. Noise should be kept to a minimum; the use of earplugs or noise-canceling headphones can be beneficial in reducing ambient noise.

3. The room temperature should be cool. A cooler surrounding will assist the athlete in falling asleep. Warm or hot surroundings add to the discomfort and are likely to disrupt normal sleep schedules. The use of a fan or air conditioner to keep temperatures cool will help to avoid unnecessary disruptions in sleep.

4. Comfort is a must for a good night's sleep. Individuals have found that using their own pillow when traveling is a great way of helping them fall asleep in unfamiliar surroundings.

Some effective strategies that an athlete can employ to help to reduce the effects of fatigue caused by sleep deprivation include napping and the strategic use of caffeine. Although sleep loss must be paid back, napping can be a very effective short-term strategy to help the athlete prolong focus and attention when sleep deprived. The recommended amount of nap time is between 30 and 60 minutes; however, if an athlete can get more than 60 minutes of needed sleep, it is highly recommended that he or she do so. A 30- to 60-minute nap can prolong mental performance for approximately 2 hours. If the athlete has an important mental task to perform immediately after napping, then the 30 to 60 minutes is advisable, as any longer napping can produce a sense of grogginess that may last for up to 20 minutes or more on waking.

Caffeine is a central-nervous stimulant and has the capacity to increase mental focus, reduce physical and mental fatigue, and improve reaction time. Athletes should use caffeine *only* when needed and should not consume it indiscriminately throughout the day. The correct use of caffeine has also been demonstrated to improve athletic performance. After 24 hours of continuous sleep deprivation, caffeine consumed at the right time in the right amounts has been scientifically proven to prolong mental performance for approximately 3 additional hours (see Question 97). Caffeine should not be consumed within 5 hours before bedtime, as it can interfere with sleep.

Sleep is vital to athletes' success both on and off the field. Athletes should try to get a minimum of 8 hours of sleep per night to ensure optimal recovery and performance. If 8 hours is difficult to get at one time, an athlete should try to squeeze in naps throughout the day to help him or her catch up. Insufficient sleep can cause lapses in attention that can lead to injuries. Getting the required amount of sleep each night will help the athlete avoid making basic mistakes.

Insufficient sleep can cause lapses in attention that can lead to injuries.

Anathea C. Powell's, MD, comments:

As a general-surgery resident, I had become detrained after many sleepless nights on call. In order to get ready for Ironman, I had to make up ground very quickly in a very short window of time during a research fellowship. In order to maximize my time and effort, I turned to experts in the field of sports nutrition and exercise science. With a professional and individualized nutrition and exercise program, I found that my body composition improved and my sleep patterns became more regulated, and I saw significant performance improvements in all of my sports. I improved 83 minutes overall in my second Ironman race and gained an edge in every stage of the race.

General Exercise Concepts

What are the health benefits of regular exercise?

What are the basic principles of exercise that are needed to optimize training and performance?

Why should athletes warm up before and cool down after exercise?

More . . .

Part 2 provides athletes with step-by-step guidance to help them train smarter, reduce injury, and perform at a higher level. This section offers athletes specific guidelines and tools to measure performance and to implement effective exercise concepts to prevent the common pitfalls that athletes regularly encounter.

16. What are the health benefits of regular exercise?

Health is defined as freedom from disease. Numerous people are unaware that they are afflicted with risk factors that can lead to chronic illnesses such as heart disease, diabetes, stroke, and certain cancers. Many risk factors often have no physical symptoms (silent), and thus, they are not felt by an individual. The most significant physiological risk factors for heart disease include high blood pressure (hypertension), elevated blood lipids (cholesterol and triglycerides), and high blood sugar (hyperglycemia). Additional risk factors include smoking, obesity, and a lack of physical activity.

Quick Fact

One of every four Americans has high blood pressure.

Uncontrollable risk factors such as genetics, age, gender, and ethnicity play a significant part in the development of disease, but chronic illnesses such as heart disease and diabetes are commonly a result of individual lifestyle (poor diet, smoking, a lack of exercise, etc.). Contemporary medicine has made great strides in treating and controlling many of the chronic diseases plaguing modern society; however, this intervention comes with a hefty price tag to both the individual and the economy.

Heart disease is still the number-one killer of both men and women in Western society. Numerous studies have demonstrated that **coronary artery disease** is two to three times higher in sedentary men than physically active men; inactivity doubles a man's chances for a heart attack. Cardiorespiratory exercise done three or more times per week for 30 to 60 minutes at a moderate intensity has been proven to lower the risk of heart disease. Greater benefits can be experienced with a higher frequency and duration, meaning more than three times per week and longer than 30 minutes.

Coronary artery disease

Progressive narrowing of the coronary arteries.

Quick Fact

500,000 Americans die from heart disease every year.

The health benefits of regular exercise include reduced total blood lipids and blood pressure, improved lipid profiles, weight management, and a strong heart and circulatory system.

1. Reduced **blood lipid profiles**: Studies have shown that regular exercise (cardiorespiratory and resistance training) can have a significant positive effect on blood lipid profiles. Both types of exercise can decrease low-density lipoprotein ("bad") cholesterol and increase high-density lipoprotein ("good") cholesterol, thus leading to an overall improvement in the low-density lipoprotein to high-density lipoprotein ratio. Additionally, the total cholesterol to high-density lipoprotein ratio improves. Low-density lipoprotein has been implicated in the development of arterial **plaque**, whereas high-density lipoprotein is known to reduce and potentially remove arterial plaque. Possessing a high total cholesterol or high low-density lipoprotein to high-density lipoprotein ratio substantially increases a person's risk for coronary artery disease. Endurance exercise has a higher positive impact on blood lipid profiles than resistance exercise.

Blood lipid profile

A blood test that determines the amount of fat in the form of cholesterol and triglyceride in the circulation.

Plaque

A build-up of lipids (fats) in the arteries of the heart that reduces blood flow.

General Exercise Concepts

Systole

The contraction phase of the heart that ejects blood into the circulatory system.

Diastole

A resting phase of the heart where blood refills the chambers of the heart.

Vascular resistance

The resistance to blood flow that must be overcome to push blood through the circulatory system.

Lean body mass

The portion of a body's makeup that consists of fat-free mass plus the essential fats that comprise those tissues.

Metabolize

The breaking down of carbohydrates, proteins, and fats into smaller units; reorganizing those units as tissue building blocks or as energy sources; and eliminating waste products of the processes.

Insulin

A naturally occurring hormone secreted by the cells of the pancreas in response to increased levels of glucose in the blood. The hormone acts to regulate the metabolism of glucose, fats, and proteins.

2. Reduced blood pressure: Regular exercise has been shown to reduce blood pressure in hypertensive individuals. The effect is more pronounced in those who have moderate hypertension compared with individuals with severe hypertension. Average blood pressure decreases of 5 mm Hg **systole** and 7 mm Hg **diastole** have been confirmed in persons suffering from mild hypertension. Although the physiological basis for the decrease in blood pressure resulting from endurance exercise is still unknown, it is theorized that endurance exercise may help to reduce **vascular resistance**. Active and fit individuals have been shown to be less susceptible to developing hypertension.

3. Weight management: Exercise promotes weight loss and helps to maintain **lean body mass**. Regular exercise (aerobic and anaerobic) in conjunction with a moderate reduction in calorie intake is an effective method for losing and maintaining weight. Exercise can help to **metabolize** glucose more efficiently from the circulation by increasing **insulin** sensitivity in the cells. This improved sensitivity helps to remove excess blood glucose for entry into the cells where it is stored as glycogen or immediately oxidized for energy. Evidence exists that demonstrates the effects of exercise on stress reduction and smoking cessation.

4. Strong heart and circulatory system: Chronic aerobic exercise has distinct anatomical and physiological effects on the human heart. Some of the more favorable changes from exercise include larger coronary arteries for better circulation, greater pumping capacity because of increased contractility, and a larger left ventricle for ejecting more blood per beat throughout the body. All of these positive changes to the heart make it stronger, more efficient, and less susceptible to a heart attack.

Even though exercise is not the universal panacea to all diseases, it can have a profound effect on reducing or eliminating some of the more insidious risk factors associated with certain chronic illnesses. Exercise has been shown through research to reduce total blood lipids and blood pressure, improve lipid profiles, control weight, and strengthen the heart and circulatory system. Anyone considering beginning an exercise program should make sure that he or she has first been given the green light by his or her physician. Consulting with a qualified and experienced exercise physiologist and registered dietitian is advisable to ensure that the program is scientifically based and safe.

Exercise has been shown through research to reduce total blood lipids and blood pressure, improve lipid profiles, control weight, and strengthen the heart and circulatory system.

General Exercise Concepts

17. What are the basic principles of exercise that are needed to optimize training and performance?

Athletes who are serious about their training and competition must ensure that they are optimally prepared by using the most current scientific methods that will allow for maximal adaptations and performance while reducing susceptibility to overtraining and injury.

In order for athletes to train and compete at the highest possible level, they must pay careful attention to scientifically sound and effective exercise strategies and principles. A well-designed exercise program, aerobic or anaerobic, should incorporate four general training principles: (1) specificity, (2) progression, (3) variation, and (4) overload.

Specificity is a training principle that necessitates an athlete to train specifically for the sport or activity. The training program incorporates the physiological requirements for the activity, including the musculoskeletal,

Specificity

A training principle that necessitates an athlete to specifically train for the sport or activity.

Respiratory
Includes airways, lungs, and respiratory muscles that allow gas exchange.

cardiovascular, **respiratory**, energy, and neuromuscular systems of the body. Training should include motor patterns that replicate the activity's movements to ensure maximum transferability and adaptation. If an athlete fails to integrate specificity into his or her training, he or she will most likely compromise his or her performance. For example, a high jumper would be best served by incorporating sport-specific movements, such as jump squats, plyometric drills, or power cleans, into his or her training program. These specific movements would prepare the jumper more effectively for competition than non–sport-specific movements. Examples of non–sport-specific movements for this athlete include endurance running, leg extensions, or bench press; these movements have little transferability to the actual activity.

Progression
A principle that requires an athlete's training program to be progressively advanced over time to ensure improvement (peaking) and reduce injury or burnout.

Progression is a principle that requires an athlete's training program to be progressively advanced over time to ensure improvement (peaking) and reduce injury or burnout. An athlete should be monitored carefully during his or her prescribed workouts to determine when training loads need to be increased or decreased. For example, a discus thrower would have a detailed strength training program designed for an entire training year. The program would be broken into specific cycles (see Question 21) that would incorporate gradual increases in workload throughout the season. If an athlete decided to leap ahead of the program, breaking the designed progression, in all likelihood, the athlete would find himself or herself peaking prematurely and missing the opportunity to compete at his or her best.

Variation
Comes from changing workloads, exercises, or both.

Variation comes from changing workloads, exercises, or both. Varying the workloads (weight lifted, sets, or repetitions) is intended to prevent overtraining.

An athlete cannot work on strength all of the time, as this can lead to injury and burnout. Regular fluctuations must be built into the program to include changes in the volume and intensity of the training. Some days would incorporate strength, some strength endurance, and others power to allow for adequate recovery and maximal adaptation. Changing exercises frequently can help to reduce boredom, improve fitness and performance, and stimulate renewed physiological adaptations through a multitude of diverse ranges of motion and planes of movement.

Overload is applied to an athlete's training program to ensure continued improvement. For overload to be effective, it must exceed an athlete's current capacity. After an athlete has adapted to a particular training load, that training load must be increased to create a stronger stimulus and further adaptation. If an athlete is not provided with a significant enough overload, further improvements in the physiological systems of the body will cease, and the athlete will plateau in his or her performance. The training load is usually increased by a definite percentage each week to allow for proper adaptation. Three training variables are manipulated to provide overload to the body's systems: (1) frequency, (2) duration, and (3) intensity.

Overload
A method of training that requires the physiological systems of the body to be increasingly stressed to ensure continued improvement.

Frequency is defined as the number of training sessions per week. To maximize performance in long-distance running, an athlete would need to train between three and five times per week. For a strength athlete, training can range between two and five sessions per week, depending on the sport. The training cycle usually determines the frequency of training and should be carefully manipulated to allow for maximal recovery, adaptation, and continued improvement.

Frequency
The number of training sessions per week.

General Exercise Concepts

Duration of training will vary according to the athlete's sport and training cycle. Athletes in the pre-season phase of training (getting ready to compete) will spend less time exercising during each session because **training intensity** will be very high. Conversely, the off-season phase will generally involve longer training sessions with low to very low intensity.

Intensity is probably the single most important variable, as it provides the required stimulus (overload) necessary for increasing performance. Intensity can come in the form of increasing the resistance lifted, working at a higher heart rate, or reducing the recovery time between sets of an exercise. Athletes engaged in strength training programs usually determine intensity based on the repetition maximum. For example, a hammer thrower may work between 60% and 100% of a one-repetition maximum for a particular exercise depending on the athlete's training cycle. For this athlete, **training volume** is usually high at the beginning of the training year, and training intensity is low—between 60% and 70% of the repetition maximum. Going into the in-season, training intensity can increase to between 85% and 97% of the repetition maximum. A runner, for example, may begin his or her seasonal training runs at 60% of his or her VO_2 max (see Question 27) for longer distances. As the season progresses, training intensities can reach 85% or higher of the VO_2 max while significantly decreasing training distance. During the latter stages of the season, a runner may alternate days of low-, moderate-, and high-intensity training to ensure maximum recovery and performance.

The basic principles of exercise were designed to help athletes improve performance, reduce injuries, and avoid overtraining. With correct application, an athlete should experience all of the positive benefits, simultaneously ensuring a long and healthy athletic career.

18. Why should athletes warm up before and cool down after exercise?

Warming up before exercise and cooling down after exercise are imperative to an athlete, helping to reduce injury, enhance performance, and promote recovery. Many athletes overlook these stages of exercise, as they do not feel that they have the time or even understand the benefits of warming up or cooling down. To profit from a thorough warm-up and cool-down, an athlete must spend at least 10 minutes before workout and 5 minutes after workout stretching the major muscle groups and joints of the body.

There are two methods of warming up: dynamic and specific.

1. A dynamic warm-up should consist of ten minutes of light exercise that involves the entire body, using both major and minor muscle groups. The warm-up should commence with five minutes of light jogging, stationary cycling, or jumping jacks, followed by dynamic muscle movements. These movements can include walking lunges, backward running, lateral shuffling, one- and two-legged hops, and walking with alternating toe touches. The purpose behind the dynamic warm-up is to increase heart rate and blood flow to the working muscles and joints, raise muscle temperature, improve muscle elasticity and plasticity, and increase respiratory rate and change joint fluid viscosity. As muscle temperature increases, joint flexibility improves, helping to reduce the athlete's susceptibility to injury.

General Exercise Concepts

2. A specific warm-up should consist of five minutes or more of sport-specific movements and stretches that simulate muscle and joint actions of the sport. For example, a basketball or volleyball player would spend time on his or her shoulder and hip muscles and joints by doing light jumping, spiking, and lay-up and shooting drills, and a baseball player would concentrate on specific throwing and upper-torso rotational movements. The purpose behind a specific warm-up is to increase functional capacity, improving sport-specific performance. An athlete, whatever the sport, needs to take the time to work on sport-specific warm-ups to ensure maximal efficiency and injury reduction.

After an intense training session or competition, an athlete must take five minutes to cool-down properly.

Venous return

The transportation of blood from the cells through the veins back to the heart.

Syncope

A sudden drop in blood pressure that causes dizziness and possible fainting.

After an intense training session or competition, an athlete must take 5 minutes to cool-down properly. The cool-down phase should involve a gradual reduction in the intensity of exercise, followed by stretching (flexibility) exercises (see Question 19). For example, at the end of a workout, a runner should reduce his or her running intensity to a light jog and then to a walk to prevent blood from pooling in his or her lower extremities. Light jogging and walking after exercise aid in **venous return**. Venous return promotes blood flow back to the heart and lungs because of the muscles contracting against the veins. This venous return helps the athlete to recover faster and reduces the potential for **syncope** (decreased blood flow to the brain), which can cause dizziness or fainting.

Athletes of all ages and abilities should take the time to learn and apply warm-ups and cool-downs to their training programs. A warm-up can help to reduce injury, improve performance, and ready the body for the rigors of the sport, whereas a cool-down can help the athlete recover faster and prevent the possibility of lightheadedness and fainting. Athletes need to ensure that the warm-up is not too intense, as it may interfere with their performance by causing premature fatigue. During the cool-down phase, an athlete should bring his or her heart rate down to less than 110 beats per minute to ensure proper recovery.

This is an example of a typical warm-up and cool-down for a baseball player:

A. Dynamic warm-up (10 minutes)
   1. Light jogging—100 meters
   2. Light jogging with giant forward arm circle—100 meters
   3. Light jogging with giant backward arm circles—100 meters
   4. Side shuffle with lateral arm raises—100 meters
   5. Carioca—100 meters
B. Sport-specific warm-up (5 to 8 minutes)
   1. Walking lunges with alternating upper-body twists (can use 2- to 4-pound medicine ball)—1 for 50 yards (see a and b)

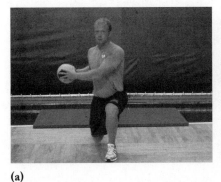
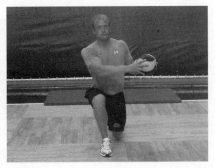

(a)   (b)

2. In-place two-legged hops—1 for 30 seconds (see c, d, and e)

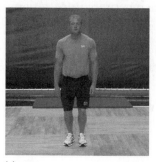

(c) start

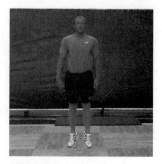

(d) jump

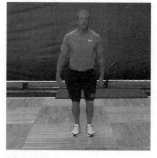

(e) finish

3. Opposite leg to opposite hand kicks—1 for 50 yards (switch legs) (see f)

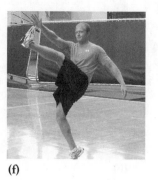

(f)

4. Light medicine ball (2 pound) throws with partner (see g and h) or wall (see i and j)—1 for 30 seconds (each arm)

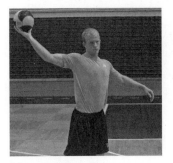

(g) preparing to throw

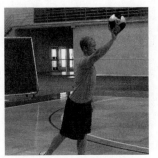

(h) throwing

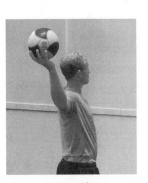

(i) preparing to throw

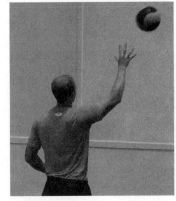

(j) throwing

C. Cool-down (5 to 8 minutes)

1. Very light walking or jogging—2 to 3 minutes
2. Seated hamstring stretches—3 for 20 to 30 seconds each (see k)

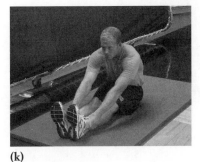

(k)

3. Shoulder stretches—3 for 20 to 30 seconds each (see l)

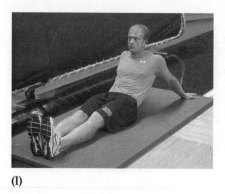

(l)

4. Groin stretches—3 for 20 to 30 seconds each (see m)

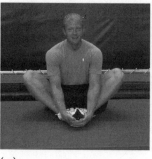

(m)

5. Thigh stretches—3 for 20 to 30 seconds, each leg (see n)

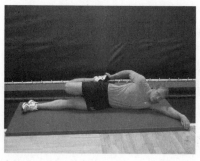

(n)

19. How can I improve my flexibility?

Flexibility is the range of motion about a joint. It is an important component of all sports; thus, athletes should work on their flexibility year round (before, during, and after the season). Athletes can improve their flexibility by incorporating three to four stretching sessions per week into their training schedule. Conversely, flexibility can deteriorate with periods of inactivity, leading to an increase in susceptibility to serious injury.

Flexibility is influenced by factors such as age, gender, activity level, and joint and tissue structure. As athletes age, the joints and surrounding tissue structures become more rigid and lose much of their elasticity, causing a decrease in range of motion. This decreased flexibility is generally the result of **fibrosis**, a condition in which fibrous connective tissue replaces muscle fibers. Females tend to have more flexibility than males because of possible structural and anatomical differences and hormonal influences. Less active individuals are inclined to have a lower level of flexibility than more active individuals. Additionally, there are inherent joint and tissue structure differences (joint capsules, tendons, ligaments, and skin) between individuals that result in varying levels of flexibility. Certain individuals have higher elasticity and plasticity components to their connective tissue, making them more flexible.

Flexibility can be attained during the warm-up and cool-down parts of a workout. After the dynamic warm-up, when muscle temperature is higher, an athlete should spend at least 5 minutes working on his or her flexibility (see Question 18). Stretching before exercise can help to reduce injuries and increase performance through enhanced elasticity of muscles, tendons, and joint range of motion and functional ability.

Flexibility

The range of motion about a joint.

Fibrosis

A condition in which fibrous connective tissue replaces muscle fibers.

General Exercise Concepts

After exercise, the muscles are warm, allowing the elastic components within the muscles and tendons to be easily stretched; warm muscles are able to stretch to greater lengths. The cool-down phase is considered to be the optimal time to maximize flexibility.

There are two recommended stretching techniques that improve flexibility: active stretching and passive stretching. An **active stretch** occurs when an athlete applies the force for the stretch. For example, the seated hamstring and lower back stretch requires the athlete to lean his or her upper torso to his or her lower torso and hold for a period of time. The **passive stretch** requires the assistance of a device or person to apply the force for the stretch.

Stretching can be subdivided into four basic stretch techniques: static, dynamic, ballistic, and proprioceptive neuromuscular facilitation.

1. **Static stretching** is often referred to as the stretch–hold technique. The athlete begins the stretch by moving the joint and muscle through a range of motion until the stretch sensation is felt in the belly of the muscle. The stretch is then held for 20 to 30 seconds followed by a relaxation period of a few seconds. The stretch is repeated for two more repetitions (trying to increase the range of motion each time) using the same technique. The athlete should avoid stretching the muscle too intensely, as this could lead to injury. Static stretching is a very effective method for increasing flexibility and is generally considered to be safe.

2. **Dynamic stretching** is a method of stretching using sport-specific movements to increase flexibility.

Active stretch

When an athlete applies the force for the stretch.

Passive stretch

Requires the use of a device or person to apply the force for the stretch.

Static stretching

Referred to as the stretch-hold technique. It begins by moving the joint and muscle through a range of motion until the stretch sensation is felt in the belly of the muscle.

Dynamic stretching

A method of stretching using sports-specific movements to increase flexibility.

This type of stretching helps to prepare an athlete for the movement patterns of his or her sport by stretching the involved muscles, tendons, and joints. For example, a pitcher in baseball could use stretch bands (rubber tubing) to simulate his or her throwing technique and/or actual ball throwing that gradually increases in intensity during each consecutive throw.

3. **Ballistic stretching** is often referred to as the bounce technique. The movement is rapid with no hold (bouncing) at the end of the stretch. The muscle is stretched quickly, returned to its original position rapidly, and then stretched again. Ballistic stretching has the potential to cause serious injury and should be avoided. During ballistic stretching, the muscle is never allowed to relax, which creates a stretch reflex in the muscle, causing it to tighten; this is counterproductive to the purpose of stretching. An example of a ballistic stretch is the standing toe touch. The athlete stands with his or her legs slightly apart and tries to touch his or her toes by bouncing up and down in rapid succession for a period of time. If an athlete has a pre-existing back or hamstring injury, the potential for further injury using this stretch is high.

> **Ballistic stretching**
>
> Often called the bounce technique; the movement is rapid with no hold at the end of the stretch.

4. **Proprioceptive neuromuscular facilitation** is often referred to as the stretch–hold–contract technique. Performance of this method of stretching usually requires a partner with a certain level of expertise. The proprioceptive neuromuscular facilitation method has been demonstrated to be a superior technique for developing flexibility, as it prolongs muscle relaxation after each stretch. There are three different types of proprioceptive neuromuscular facilitation stretching; the most commonly used

> **Proprioceptive neuromuscular facilitation**
>
> Often referred to as the stretch–hold–contract technique. This method of stretching usually requires a partner with a certain level of expertise to perform.

and effective method is the hold–relax–contract technique. An example of the hold–relax–contract technique for a hamstring stretch requires the athlete to lie flat on his or her back. A partner would then raise one of athlete's legs passively until a slightly uncomfortable muscle stretch was felt in the hamstring. The athlete is required to keep the leg straight and the knee locked during the entire stretch. The partner instructs the athlete to apply downward force against the partner's hand with the partner resisting the leg from moving. The **isometric** contraction on the leg is held for 6 seconds and then allowed to relax for a few seconds. The partner then applies a second passive stretch (greater than the initial stretch) and should be held for a period of 30 seconds. This stretching technique can be applied to most joints of the body and is a very effective method for improving flexibility.

Isometric

Muscular contraction resulting in no change in the muscle's length.

Flexibility can be acquired rapidly and has the potential to increase performance and reduce injury.

Flexibility is a crucial part of an athlete's sports enhancement program. Flexibility can be acquired rapidly and has the potential to increase performance and reduce injury. To increase flexibility, stretching is recommended to be done after exercise when the athlete's muscles and tendons are warm and most receptive to being stretched. Long periods of inactivity can decrease flexibility quickly and should be avoided.

20. What is the difference between slow- and fast-twitch muscle fibers, and what role do they play during exercise?

Athletes' muscles are not uniform throughout their body. Human skeletal muscle is comprised of two different types of muscle fiber, slow twitch (type 1) and fast twitch (type 2), in approximately equal amounts.

Fast-twitch fibers can be further subdivided into type 2a and type 2b fibers.

Slow-twitch muscle fibers have a reddish appearance because of their high **myoglobin** content and have a relatively slow contractile force. They have a high **mitochondria** content and are surrounded by numerous blood vessels (capillaries) that bring oxygen and nutrient-rich blood into the muscle. Type 1 muscle fibers produce energy aerobically (in the presence of oxygen) and are very efficient at producing ATP (energy needed for the contraction and relaxation of muscle) from the oxidation of fats and carbohydrates; thus, they are recruited quickly, are remarkably fatigue resistant, and are used exclusively during endurance events (such as marathon running and long-distance cycling).

Fast-twitch fibers, on the other hand, are whitish in color, contract three to four times faster than slow-twitch fibers, have a low endurance capacity, and are considerably larger than slow-twitch fibers. Type 2 muscle fibers generate most of their ATP energy anaerobically (without oxygen) from carbohydrates (**glycolysis**). Fast-twitch muscle fibers are recruited during high-intensity exercise such as sprinting and weight training. There are, however, distinct physiological differences between the type 2a and type 2b fast-twitch muscle fibers.

Type 2a muscle fibers perform similarly to both fast- and slow-twitch fibers; they have a relatively higher blood flow capacity, a higher capillary density, and a higher mitochondrial content than type 2b fibers, and they are relatively fatigue resistant. Type 2a muscle fibers have some capacity for oxidative metabolism (utilization of fats and carbohydrates for energy).

Myoglobin
Found mainly in muscle tissue; serves as a storage site for oxygen.

Mitochondria
Powerhouses of the cell that burn carbohydrates, fats, and proteins for energy.

Glycolysis
Breakdown of glucose into energy.

General Exercise Concepts

They are considered to be an intermediate fiber that is used extensively during activities of moderate to high intensity, lasting only a few minutes, such as a 1-mile run or a 400-meter swim (middle-distance events).

Type 2b fibers have a very low blood supply, a low mitochondrial content, and a low capillary density, and they fatigue rapidly during exercise. Type 2b fibers are recruited during very intense exercise, such as a 100-meter sprint or a 50-meter sprint swim, and produce energy exclusively through anaerobic metabolism of carbohydrates. The amount of force generated by type 2b muscle fibers is considerably greater than by type 2a, and in essence, a type 2b muscle fiber is a power fiber.

During exhaustive exercise, such as marathon running, the body preferentially recruits slow-twitch muscle fibers first. At some undetermined point, slow-twitch fibers begin to fatigue from glycogen depletion. The reduction in glycogen content eventually forces the body to transition to the fast-twitch type 2a fibers to maintain performance. When type 2a fibers exhaust their energy stores, the body finally activates the type 2b fibers to keep the muscles fueled. When the type 2b fibers are glycogen depleted, the body experiences volitional fatigue ("bonking"), which causes a significant drop in performance (see **Table 4**).

The ratio of fast-twitch to slow-twitch fibers appears to be genetically determined at a very young age, possibly the first few years of life. Fiber distribution is inherited and cannot be significantly altered through training. Studies completed on identical twins clearly demonstrate inheritance as a major factor in determining fiber type and distribution; results prove that their fiber types are almost indistinguishable.

Table 4   Attributes of Slow-Twitch and Fast-Twitch Muscle Fibers

		Fiber Type	
	Slow Twitch	Fast Twitch Type a	Fast Twitch Type b
Contraction speed	Slow	Moderately fast	Very fast
Duration of use	Hours	< 5 min	< 1 min
Fatigability	Low	Moderately high	High
Physical activity	Aerobic	Long anaerobic	Short anaerobic
Capillary density	High	Moderate	Low
Mitochondrial density	High	Moderately high	Low
Oxidative capacity	High	Moderately high	Low
Glycolytic capacity	Low	High	High
Major fuel storage	Triglycerides (fats)	Glycogen/Pc	Glycogen/Pc

Although fiber type cannot be significantly altered through training, recent studies now show that training may have a small but significant impact on type 1 and type 2 fibers. It has been estimated, through research, that approximately 10% of fast- and slow-twitch fibers can be altered through training. Regular strength training has been shown to shift a small percentage of type 2a muscle fibers to type 2b. Conversely, shifts of approximately 3% to 4% of type 2b fibers can be converted to type 2a fibers as a result of chronic endurance training. In addition, as an athlete ages, there appears to be an appreciable change in muscle fiber distribution, with a shift from fast-twitch to slow-twitch fibers.

An athlete's success in a particular sport is determined by several factors, including training, cardiovascular

General Exercise Concepts

function, muscle size, motivation, coaching, and muscle fiber composition. The relative percentage and distribution of type 1 and type 2 muscle fibers usually steer an athlete into a particular sport or activity. Athletes who are endowed with a higher percentage of slow-twitch fiber are more likely to gravitate to endurance-type activities, such as marathon running. Conversely, athletes endowed with a higher percentage of fast-twitch fibers are more inclined to be better at strength or power sports, such as sprinting. Athletes with almost equal ratios of type 1 and 2 fibers tend to be better at moderate- to high-intensity activities, such as the mile run. Most athletes discover what they are better suited to by experimenting with different activities at a young age. Comparatively, world-class endurance athletes have been shown to have as much as 90% or more type 1 fiber in their gastrocnemius (calf) muscles, as opposed to elite sprinters, who have only 20% to 25%; therefore, it would make little sense for an athlete suited for endurance to become a power athlete and vice versa (**Table 5**).

Table 5   Comparison of Approximate Fiber Types Based on Various Sports

Sport	Muscle	Percentage of Slow Twitch	Percentage of Fast Twitch
Marathon	Gastrocnemius (calf)	80	20
Swimming	Posterior Deltoid (rear shoulder)	65	35
Cycling	Vastus Lateralis (outer thigh)	60	40
Sprinting	Gastrocnemius (calf)	25	75
Javelin Thrower	Gastrocnemius (calf)	35	65
Sedentary	Vastus lateralis (outer thigh)	45	55

Athletes should be encouraged to develop the appropriate fiber type for their sport through a well-developed, scientifically based, sport-specific training program created by a qualified exercise specialist.

21. What is periodization? Why is it important?

For decades, athletes prepared for competition by using a trial and error approach to their training. Training was rarely scientifically based, and athletes usually experimented with a variety of approaches hoping to discover the one that was most effective. If a particular method failed to produce the desired results, athletes typically moved on to a different program. The ultimate cost of using an ad hoc approach to training frequently resulted in the athlete failing to reach his or her optimal athletic potential. Athletes often fell into the trap of training too hard too often and for too long, leading to unnecessary injuries and overtraining. As a response to this hit-or-miss approach to training, Eastern European Bloc countries began developing and using a more scientific approach to athlete preparation. The scientific method of establishing a relationship between training intensity and **volume** over time is referred to as **periodization**. This method of training is very successful at preparing and peaking athletes for competition and has become the standardized training method for athletes throughout the world.

Periodization (cycling) is a system of training that allows individual variations in program volume and intensity over a specific period of time. The relationship between intensity and volume is typically an inverse one—in other words, as intensity increases, volume decreases and vice versa (**Figure 3**). The period covers an entire training

Volume

The amount of work done during an exercise bout.

Periodization

A method of training that varies the volume and intensity of training over a period of time to prevent overtraining.

General Exercise Concepts

45

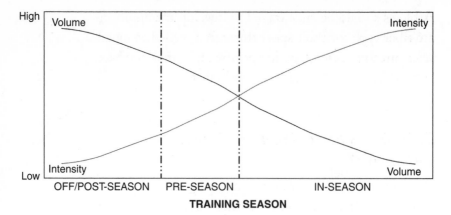

Figure 3   Relationship Between Volume and Intensity of Training.

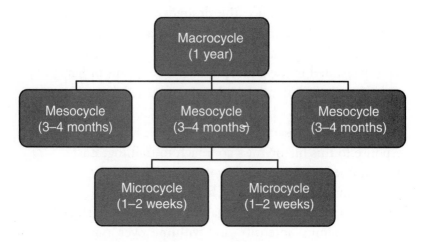

Figure 4   Annual Periodized Training Program Cycles.

year for the majority of athletes, but can be as long as 4 years for Olympic athletes. The classic periodization model (**Figure 4**) is broken into three phases: macrocycle, mesocycle, and microcycle. The first phase, macrocycle, is the longest phase and is usually a year long. This cycle spans the four seasonal periods of off-season, post-season, pre-season, and in-season. The second phase, mesocycle, can last for several months. Usually there are three or more mesocycles per macrocycle, depending on the sport and number of competitions throughout the year. The last phase, microcycle, lasts one week or more, concentrating on daily and weekly training fluctuations. There are approximately three or more microcycles per mesocycle.

The purpose behind the periodization concept is to help prevent the athlete from burning out and/or overtraining (see Question 83). Periodization necessitates that the athlete's training program consist of a period of non–sport-specific activities during the early part of the season where training volume is kept high and the intensity relatively low. As the season progresses toward competition, the athlete must change his or her exercise focus to incorporate sport-specific training with higher intensity and lower volume. This scientific approach to training reduces the potential of overtraining and simultaneously maximizes performance outcomes.

A widespread approach to a training cycle for many athletes is dividing their actual training sessions into four major periods. The period that the athlete will cover depends on what part of the season the athlete is in. The four periods include preparatory, first transition, competition, and second transition. Each period covers a specific training method.

The first period is the preparatory period and is usually the longest, covering very limited sport-specific skills. The primary emphasis during this period is to focus on a basic level of conditioning that can include very low-intensity distance running, swimming, and cycling. During the early part of this period, the athlete usually engages in basic strength training exercises that involve high-repetition loads and low resistance. This helps prepare the body for the more strenuous workouts as the period progresses. Because of the high volume of training during this stage and its effects on the athletes' time and energy stores, athletes are highly discouraged from trying to add additional training components into this period such as plyometrics or intervals. A typical resistance training program during the preparatory period would be subdivided into varying strength phases needed for success. The phases in order of importance are endurance/hypertrophy, basic strength, and strength/power. These phases are designed to build muscle, increase endurance and optimal strength, and develop sports-specific explosiveness and power (see **Table 6**). Each phase has a designated period that builds on the previous phase. As each phase progresses, training intensity and volume will increase and decrease, respectively.

Table 6   Periodized Strength Training Program Recommendations from the Preparatory to the Competition Periods

Training Phase	Intensity of % 1RM*	Volume	Sets	Repetitions
Hypertrophy/ endurance	50% to 75%	Moderate to very High	3–6	10–20
Basic strength	80% to 90%	Moderate	3–5	4–8
Maximum strength and power	75% to 95%	Low	3–5	2–5
Competition	95% to 100%	Very low	1–3	1–3
Maintenance	80% to 85%	Moderate	2–3	6–8
Active rest	Recreational activities with little to no strength training			

*1RM = one repetition maximum

The first transition period is the second stage and falls between the preparatory and competition period. This period is usually the crossover point between training intensity and volume.

The third period is the early competition period and is a very intense training phase in which the athlete concentrates heavily on sport-specific skills and game strategy. During this period, training volume is very low and intensity high, allowing the athlete to focus on peak strength and power during skill development. As the season progresses, the athlete will need to manipulate his or her training intensity and volume carefully during the weeks leading up to and during competition. This will ultimately help the athlete avoid overtraining and unnecessary injury and performance decrement. The competition season should be used principally for performance maintenance as opposed to trying to increase the athlete's capacity.

The final period is the second transition, or active rest period. During this period, the athlete unloads by spending as much as 1 to 4 weeks (depending on the sport and season) resting from the rigors of training and competition. This period is designed to help the athlete recover from injuries and the physical and mental demands of his or her sport. During this period, an athlete will engage in low-impact activities that are unrelated to his or her sport. For example, a soccer player may play volleyball or tennis during this period, allowing him or her to recover not only physically and mentally but also to help maintain his or her fitness. Athletes should try to avoid **inactive rest**, as this may lead to unwanted detraining.

Inactive rest

An extended period of inactivity.

The benefits of periodized training are well documented. Periodization helps an athlete reach peak performance through steady progressive training, and at the same time avoiding the mistakes of overtraining and possible injury. Athletes who are inexperienced in developing periodized programs should consult with a knowledgeable and qualified strength and conditioning specialist to help them design and implement a sport-specific periodized plan.

> ### Quick Fact
>
> A periodized exercise program should be complemented with a well-developed periodized nutrition program.

22. What causes muscle soreness after exercise?

Nearly everyone can claim to have experienced some type of muscle soreness after engaging in exercise. Muscle soreness is commonly referred to as delayed-onset muscle soreness. Delayed-onset muscle soreness describes a phenomenon of muscle pain or muscle stiffness that generally occurs 12 to 48 hours after exercise. This usually occurs in individuals who are unaccustomed to exercising, make sudden increases in training intensity and/or volume after periods of extended inactivity, or are immobilized because of injury.

The pain is not uncommon and is usually necessary to help the body adapt to greater workloads leading to improved strength, endurance, and muscle development. Typically, the pain gets progressively worse within the first 48 hours after activity and generally subsides within 4 to 7 days, depending on how much damage is done to the muscle.

Delayed-onset muscle soreness is thought to result from tiny tears occurring in the membranes of the muscle fibers. The amount of damage is dependent on certain factors such as how hard, how long, and what type of exercise an athlete has engaged in. When the muscle fibers are damaged, inflammation (swelling) occurs and puts pressure on the surrounding nerves, leading to pain and tenderness. In contrast to popular belief, delayed-onset muscle soreness is not the result of lactic acid left in the muscle, as the majority of lactic acid is usually removed within a few minutes after exercise. The bulk of muscle damage is caused by **eccentric** muscle actions. Eccentric muscle actions involve movements that cause the muscle to contract while lengthening. Examples of eccentric muscle actions include going down stairs, downhill running, and the lowering of weights in the gym.

An effective way to mitigate delayed-onset muscle soreness is prevention. The most reliable method to eliminate or reduce the effects of delayed-onset muscle soreness is to begin unaccustomed exercise slowly, with very light workloads, and gradually build up to higher intensities and durations over time. This progressive training method has been demonstrated to be the most beneficial in helping to reduce delayed-onset muscle soreness. Other methods for reducing delayed-onset muscle soreness may include a thorough warm-up before exercise, followed by a cool-down with gentle stretching after exercise.

After muscle tissue damage has occurred, one can do little to stop the damage process and the accompanying soreness; however, a few tips that can be applied to help reduce some of the discomfort of delayed-onset muscle soreness. Some athletes have found relief from using ice baths, massage, very light exercise, light stretching, post-workout nutrition, and the use of certain over-the-counter pain relievers. In addition, a few research studies have even reported that a strong foundation in Yoga can help. More recent studies have shown promise with

General Exercise Concepts

Eccentric

Movements that cause the muscle to contract while lengthening. Examples of eccentric muscle actions include going down stairs, downhill running, and the lowering of weights in the gym.

The most reliable method to eliminate or reduce the effects of delayed-onset muscle soreness is to begin unaccustomed exercise slowly, with very light workloads, and gradually build up to higher intensities and durations over time.

Anticatabolic substance

A nutritional compound that slows the breakdown process in the body (catabolism), thus tilting the metabolic balance toward increased tissue building (anabolism).

Whey protein

A biproduct of cheese manufacturing. It is a short peptide-bonded protein and is rapidly digested and absorbed into the circulation (bloodstream). Whey protein is found in yogurt and cottage cheese (the liquid on the surface of the product before it is mixed).

Exercise-induced rhabdomyolysis

A condition resulting from an acute skeletal muscle injury that causes the muscle cell membrane to break open, spilling its contents into the circulation.

Compartment syndrome

Increased pressure caused by inflammation within a muscle compartment of the body, impairing its blood supply.

certain **anticatabolic substances** (caffeine, hydroxy-methylbuterate [HMB], **whey protein**); however, these studies are not yet conclusive, and recommendations cannot be made with the limited data currently available.

23. How can I tell if I have exercise-induced rhabdomyolysis or delayed-onset muscle soreness?

Exercise-induced rhabdomyolysis is a rare but potentially serious (and life-threatening) condition that is generally brought on by too much exercise at one time. It affects people of all ages, races, fitness levels, and genders. Most exercise-induced rhabdomyolysis cases have been reported in military, law enforcement, and fire department personnel because of a vigilant documentation process. Cases in the public sector are generally not documented or reported; therefore, the statistics are unknown.

Exercise-induced rhabdomyolysis results from an acute skeletal muscle injury that causes the muscle cell membrane to break open, spilling its contents into the circulation. Some of the cellular debris includes myoglobin, creatine kinase, potassium, and other various intracellular contents. Abnormally high amounts of this cellular debris can lead to serious health issues such as renal (kidney) failure, cardiac dysrhythmias, **compartment syndrome**, and even death.

In determining whether an athlete has exercise-induced rhabdomyolysis (versus delayed-onset muscle soreness), the diagnosis consists of three distinct details:

1. Swollen and severe incapacitating pain in the muscles
2. Elevated creatine kinase levels in the blood
3. Myoglobin in the urine

This triad of symptoms is found in exercise-induced rhabdomyolysis only and not in delayed-onset muscle soreness. The mild to moderate muscle soreness that accompanies delayed-onset muscle soreness usually dissipates within 48 hours with no further complications, whereas athletes diagnosed with exercise-induced rhabdomyolysis typically experience very painful muscles with limited range of motion during flexion and extension. The muscle is tender to the touch and is usually swollen.

Creatine kinase levels in normal muscle range between 55 and 170 U/L. In severe cases of exercise-induced rhabdomyolysis, ranges from 10,000 to 300,000 U/L have been reported, whereas creatine kinases levels in delayed-onset muscle soreness rarely get over a few thousand units per liter. Creatine kinase levels normally peak in the bloodstream within 24 to 36 hours.

During exercise-induced rhabdomyolysis, myoglobin (a reddish muscle protein that is responsible for carrying oxygen from the cell membrane to the mitochondria) levels in the blood reach such high levels that myoglobin gets carried into the urine. If left untreated in the urine, myoglobin will start to collect in the kidneys and has a high potential to cause renal failure. Dark-brown or rust color urine is one of the first signs that an athlete may be experiencing rhabdomyolysis. This change in urine color is a definite indication that myoglobin has spilled into the urine. If an athlete experiences this symptom, he or she should seek medical help immediately because as many as one third of all patients who have rhabdomyolysis experience acute renal failure.

Several of the predisposing risk factors for developing exercise-induced rhabdomyolysis include the following:

1. A rapid increase in intensity or duration of demanding physical activity
2. Activity that requires a heavy eccentric (muscle lengthening) component
3. Dehydration
4. Exercising in high heat and or humidity
5. Predisposition to heat illness or previous heat injury
6. Illness (bacterial, viral)
7. Recent medication or drug use (aspirin, cholesterol-lowering medications, alcohol)
8. Genetic disorders (sickle cell trait, hypothyroidism, renal insufficiency)

The best treatment for exercise-induced rhabdomyolysis is education and prevention. Athletes should remember the principles of training (see Question 17) when designing an exercise program. Exercise should be progressive with gradual increases in the workload over time to ensure maximum adaptation and recovery. Athletes should try to avoid exercising during high temperatures and humid conditions. If this is not possible, then an athlete needs to be educated on proper **acclimatization** techniques, as well as the correct timing for and type and amounts of foods and fluids needed to optimize performance, enhance recovery, and avoid unnecessary injuries (rhabdomyolysis) (see Part Three). Athletes who are unfamiliar with these strategies should seek the help of a licensed sports dietitian, a qualified exercise physiologist, and/or a strength and conditioning specialist.

Acclimatization

A process in which the body undergoes physiological adjustments or adaptations to changes in environmental conditions such as altitude, temperature, and humidity. The physiological changes enable the body to function better in the new climate.

■ *Case Study*

Al, a 22-year-old healthy male Marine infantry soldier, reported to his primary care clinic with complaints of severe muscle and joint pain with an inability to flex or extend his arms and dark, cola-colored urine after participating in a **fad exercise** program. The previous day Al was required to perform multiple sets of body weight chin-ups. The temperature during his workout was 105°F and 80% humidity. Al added two additional sets of chin-ups to his usual workout that day. Each additional set was done to exhaustion with every eccentric contraction being completed as slow as possible. Al also claimed that he had not consumed much fluid before or during the workout.

On initial examination, it was suspected that Al was possibly suffering from exercise-induced rhabdomyolysis. Laboratory tests were ordered, and results revealed that Al's creatine kinase levels were over 70,000 U/L and myoglobin was in the urine. Al was then admitted to the local inpatient facility for observation. During his stay, intravenous fluids were administered, and laboratory values were monitored. Laboratory values returned to normal after 4 days, and Al was discharged with the advice to make an appointment with the licensed sports dietitian and strength and conditioning specialist.

The visit with the sports dietitian revealed that Al was not drinking sufficient fluids (water and sports beverages), and thus, a specific drinking plan was designed to help him optimally hydrate (see Question 57). In addition, the sports dietitian educated Al about the common signs and symptoms of dehydration and the system for measuring and replacing fluids lost from the body (see Question 64). Within a few weeks of implementing the sports dietitian's advice, Al noticed a substantial improvement in his exercise capacity and hydration status.

Al also made an appointment to see the strength and conditioning specialist to help devise a scientifically based strength program. The conditioning specialist

Fad exercise
Exercise programs or ideas that promise to deliver quick gains with minimal or maximal effort.

General Exercise Concepts

educated Al on what and how to implement the basic principles of exercise into a periodized format to help prevent overtraining situations and the risk of injury (see Question 21). Over the next month, Al noticed significant strength gains from his program with less time spent in the gym. Al was lucky that this condition was relatively mild in comparison to more severe cases that usually require longer hospitalization, rehabilitation, and pharmacological intervention.

24. What causes cramps and/or stitches during exercise?

Cramps

Painful involuntary muscle contractions that usually occur in the body's lower-extremity muscles (calves, hamstrings, quadriceps).

Stitches

Similar to cramps. They occur in the upper body typically between the lower ribs and pelvis.

Cramps are painful involuntary muscle contractions that usually occur in the body's lower-extremity muscles (calves, hamstrings, and quadriceps). The onset of cramps is usually quick and can last from seconds to minutes. **Stitches** are similar to cramps and occur in the upper body, typically between the lower ribs and pelvis. The pain is localized and frequently triggered by repetitive movements by the upper torso such as in running and/or swimming. The exact cause of a stitch is unknown. Some of the common causes and potential remedies of cramps and stitches are listed in **Table 7**.

If an athlete experiences a stitch or a cramp while exercising, he or she should terminate exercise. Some immediate treatments for cramps include massage, stretching, and ice application. An effective treatment for stitches involves the athlete bending over at the waist at the same time pushing on the irritated area while taking deep breaths.

Cramps and stitches most often are not signs of a serious medical condition, but if athletes are experiencing reoccurring episodes, they should consult with a healthcare provider.

Table 7   Common Causes and Potential Remedies for Cramps and Stitches

Causes	Remedies
Dehydration	Ensure adequate fluid consumption before, during, and after exercise
Electrolyte imbalances	Consume beverages that are formulated with electrolytes
Consumption of a low-carbohydrate diet	Consume at least 50% to 60% of the diet as carbohydrate
Fatigued muscles (from low levels of fitness, working at high intensity/workloads, or inadequate recovery)	Ensure that the athlete develops a progressive exercise program and gets plenty of rest between workouts
Consuming a meal/snack close to exercise	Consume a small meal or snack at least 30 to 60 minutes before exercise
Consuming a meal/snack that is high in fat or protein before exercise	Consume foods that are low in fat and protein before exercise
Sudden increases in intensity or duration of exercise	Increase exercise intensity gradually over time
Use of supplements (including creatine)	Avoid supplements
Infrequent participation in exercise	Regular exercise at least three to five times per week

25. What is rating of perceived exertion?

The **rating of perceived exertion** (RPE) scale has become a useful tool for athletes to use in determining their exercise intensity. It is a relatively easy and convenient method to help athletes rate how hard they are working during exercise. RPE is based on a scale that is often referred to as the **Borg scale**. The scale has a numerical value attached to it, increasing by 1 unit starting at 6 and ending at 20. A rating of 6 (no exertion at all)

Rating of perceived exertion (RPE)

Often referred to as the Borg scale (see Borg scale).

Borg scale

Is also known as the Rating of Perceived Exertion scale. The scale has a numerical value attached to it, increasing by 1 unit starting at 6 and ending at 20. A rating of 6 (no exertion at all) would be given by someone relaxing, whereas a rating of 20 (maximal exertion) could be given by an athlete at the end of a hard sprint. The scale is an effective tool in helping athletes to select an exercise intensity without having to use a heart rate monitor.

Research has demonstrated clearly that intensity is the most important exercise variable when it comes to developing higher levels of cardiorespi-ratory fitness.

would be given by someone relaxing, whereas a rating of 20 (maximal exertion) could be given by an athlete at the end of a hard sprint. The Borg scale can be an effective tool in helping athletes to select an exercise intensity without having to use a **heart rate monitor** (see Question 26). Research has demonstrated clearly that intensity is the most important exercise variable when it comes to developing higher levels of cardiorespiratory fitness.

Borg Scale

6 No exertion at all

7 Very, very light

8

9 Very light

10

11 Fairly light

12

13 Somewhat hard

14

15 Hard

16

17 Very hard

18

19 Very, very hard

20 Maximal

Source: Borg, 1982.

26. Can an athlete benefit from using a heart rate monitor?

Many athletes demand a more scientific approach to their training. One instrument that has become increasingly popular among recreational as well as elite athletes is the heart rate monitor. Heart rate monitors are wireless devices that consist of a transmitter (strapped around the chest) and a watch-like receiver (worn around the wrist). Heart rate monitors are easy to use and can be purchased relatively inexpensively. The benefits of using heart rate monitors are numerous:

1. Helps to quantify the athlete's training
2. Provides feedback on the body's response to the stress of training/competition
3. Allows athletes to make adjustments to their training intensity
4. Ensures continued improvement in cardiovascular fitness
5. Reduces the potential for overtraining
6. Helps those athletes recovering from detraining or injury

27. What is VO_2 max test? What does it measure? Why is it beneficial?

The **VO_2 max test** is an accurate scientific laboratory method for measuring an athlete's **cardiorespiratory** (aerobic) capacity. The VO_2 max test determines the maximum amount of oxygen in milliliters that an athlete can consume per kilogram of body weight per minute during a graded exercise test. The test is designed to assess the three major interrelated physiological systems of the body: pulmonary (lungs), cardiovascular (heart and blood vessels), and muscular. It is

VO_2 max test

An accurate scientific laboratory method of measuring an athlete's cardiorespiratory (aerobic) capacity. The VO_2 max test determines the maximum amount of oxygen in milliliters that an athlete can consume per kilogram of body weight per minute during a graded exercise test.

Cardiorespiratory

Function of both the heart and lungs.

well documented that highly trained athletes will have higher VO_2 max capacities than untrained individuals. The athlete's increased ability to extract and use oxygen at the **cellular level** will enable him or her to train with greater intensity, simultaneously buffering the body's **lactate** production, resulting in an increased resistance to fatigue. The results of a VO_2 max test may be used in the design of an athlete's sports-specific training program and can be a reliable method of measuring the athlete's physiological improvement over time.

VO_2 max assessments are generally conducted on a treadmill, bicycle, and rowing ergometer or in a swim flume (see **Figure 5**). The VO_2 max test is a progressive test that increases in intensity over time (minutes). As the workload rises, the body's capacity to extract and use circulating oxygen will also increase until the athlete reaches a maximum threshold of consumption.

Cellular level

The smallest structure that is capable of independent functioning in an organism.

Lactate

The biproduct of cellular glucose breakdown.

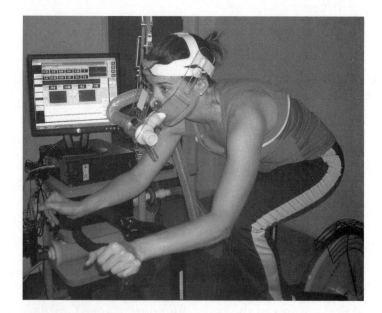

Figure 5   VO$_2$ Max Test.

After threshold is attained, further jumps in intensity will not be matched by increases in the cell's oxygen utilization. This is the athlete's upper limit, the VO_2 max. VO_2 max is expressed relative to a person's weight in ml/kg/min.

Athletes considering a VO_2 max test should be aware that the testing is exercise modality specific. In other words, biking VO_2 max data should not be used to assess running capacity and vice versa. Athletes should only be tested for their particular sport to avoid potential erroneous data being applied to their training.

Christopher's comments:

Approximately a year and a half ago I completed a 3-year sea-duty tour in the U.S. Navy and headed to shore-duty assignment. After 3 years of high-operational tempo, I found that my physical fitness level wasn't where I wanted it to be.

Now that I had the time, I wanted to get back into training, specifically for a number of adventure races coming up that summer. An opportunity presented itself to take part in a VO_2 max test in order to establish my baseline fitness level. I wasn't familiar with this test at the time, only having seen it used by Olympic athletes on a TV special during the run up to the 2008 Olympics. Frankly, I didn't think this test was geared for the "recreational athlete."

Luckily, my assessment was wrong. Although my VO_2 max numbers were not that impressive, the information garnered from the test was invaluable in tailoring my training. What I learned was that the training I was *doing was too intense and of not sufficient duration. This led to good anaerobic capability but less than optimal aerobic capability. The VO_2 max test helped map my aerobic/anaerobic threshold and give me the insight I needed to adjust my training to improve my aerobic capability.*

The difference in my race time before the test and the race I just recently ran was dramatic. I'm convinced a big part of that was due to the training plan derived from my VO_2 max test. With limited time to train, the VO_2 max test has certainly helped me train "smarter not harder."

28. Are all metabolic carts (VO_2 max assessment devices) alike?

With the advent of cheap, easy-to-use metabolic assessment systems on the market today, the availability of laboratory metabolic testing (VO_2 max) has grown considerably. Athletes today have an array of testing services available to select from as a result of these less expensive and less cumbersome systems. Unfortunately, many athletes are unaware that not all metabolic devices are created equal and subsequently may not accurately assess or measure changes in cardiorespiratory capacity. The consequence of being tested by less reliable and invalid systems could result in erroneous data being used to design an athlete's exercise program that may lead to suboptimal gains and/or possible overtraining.

In order to ensure accurate results, the athlete should ask a series of questions before considering using a VO_2 max testing facility. Top questions to consider before testing can be found in **Table 8**.

Table 8   Questions to Ask Before Choosing a Metabolic Testing Facility

Questions	Correct Answers
Is there any scientific literature that supports the machine's validity, reliability, and repeatability?	Look for legitimate information from scientific, peer-reviewed journals that provide unbiased recommendations.
What is the source of funding for the research?	Look for independent research funding that is unaffiliated with the company.
Does the metabolic cart require calibration before use?	The most accurate and reliable metabolic carts require calibration before each use; this includes gas and flow calibration, temperature, humidity, and barometric pressure.
What is the cost of the device?	Less accurate and reliable metabolic systems are relatively inexpensive (less than $5,000 to $6,000), whereas the most accurate and reliable devices are usually more than $35,000.
What breathing apparatus is used?	Two types of breathing devices are available for testing: the face mask and the mouthpiece. The mouthpiece provides a better seal, as it fits into the mouth, allowing the athlete to form a tighter seal to ensure no leakage. The face mask can be less reliable as individual faces have different contours that may prevent the mask from form fitting, thus increasing potential for leakage and data contamination.

29. What is lactate?

During very intense exercise, the development of the "burn" in muscles usually is referred to as **lactic acidosis**. This theory is still taught in many physiology courses throughout the world. To set the record straight, recent research is disputing this popular interpretation. Looking briefly at some basic physiology will help to explain one of the primary causes of muscle fatigue.

Lactic acidosis

A condition in which there is a significant accumulation of hydrogen ions in the blood and tissue, leading to muscle acidification.

General Exercise Concepts

During the demands of high-intensity exercise, the cells use a substantial amount of glucose and glycogen (stored glucose) for energy. The biproduct of cellular glucose breakdown is lactate. This increase in lactate coincides with an increase in blood and muscle acidity (hydrogen ions), which is one of the culprits of muscular fatigue; therefore, even though lactate is not responsible for the actual burn, it is an excellent indirect method of determining the level of cellular fatigue using lactate testing (see Question 30).

30. What is the lactate threshold? Why is it beneficial? How is it measured?

At rest and under steady-state exercise conditions, there is a delicate balance between the amount of blood lactate produced and the amount of blood lactate removed (metabolized) in the body. The lactate threshold is the point above which there begins an abrupt increase in lactate levels caused by an increase in exercise intensity—that is, the point in which blood lactate accumulation exceeds removal.

Lactate threshold testing

Considered by sports scientists to be one of the single most important markers of success in endurance-related activities.

Lactate threshold testing is considered by sports scientists to be one of the single most important measures of success in endurance-related activities. Determining and correctly using lactate testing data can help athletes to train and compete at the right intensities to avoid premature fatigue and/or overtraining.

The lactate threshold can be measured accurately using a reliable lactate analyzer. Lactate devices today have become more miniaturized and can be conveniently transported to the field or pool for onsite testing. To test for the lactate threshold, an athlete will be subjected to a graded exercise test either in the laboratory (bike, treadmill), on the field, or in the pool. Each endurance exercise stage lasts approximately 4 minutes, and each successive step increases in intensity challenging the athlete's energy systems. Blood lactate draws, using a finger stick, are taken at the end of each stage and evaluated and recorded on the lactate analyzer. The lactate values from each stage are plotted on a graph that corresponds to the athlete's workload. Graph analysis clearly demonstrates the point at which there is a significant increase in lactate levels (lactate threshold). Training correctly, in conjunction with regular lactate testing, can have a significant positive effect on an athlete's lactate threshold and performance.

Figures 6 and **7** depict a positive change in an athlete's lactate threshold level as a result of a 4-month lactate improvement training program designed by an exercise physiologist. The difference in lactate threshold between

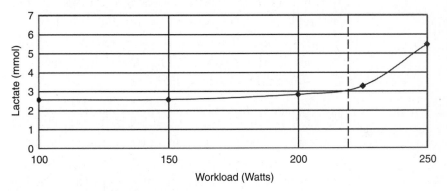

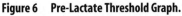

Figure 6   Pre-Lactate Threshold Graph.

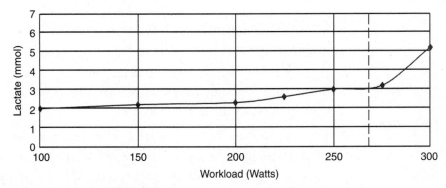

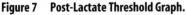

Figure 7   Post-Lactate Threshold Graph.

the pre-training and post-training program can be seen in the changes of the deflection points (see the dashed line on each graph). The data demonstrate that this athlete has improved by approximately 50 watts of power in 4 months, a significant improvement.

31. What is the better method of determining my exercise training heart rate zone?

Heart rate monitoring is the most common method used by athletes to gauge their intensity of exercise. Heart rate reflects the amount of work that the heart is performing for a particular workload. During exercise, the heart responds to increased stress by beating faster to provide necessary oxygen-rich blood to the exercising muscles. There is a lineal relationship between the workload and heart rate; as workload increases, so does heart rate. Heart rate tops out when the body achieves volitional fatigue (exhaustion) and is relatively reliable from one workout to next. This maximum heart rate value is often referred to as HRmax.

Heart rate is usually measured at the radial pulse (wrist) or carotid artery (neck). Resting heart rate is the heart rate of an athlete while at rest and varies significantly between athletes. The variability is dependent on an athlete's genetics, age, fitness level, and time of day.

1. Genetics: Some athletes are born with either a higher or lower resting heart rate.
2. Age: Resting heart rate declines with age and drops approximately one beat per minute, per year starting around the age of 15 years.
3. Fitness: Resting heart rate generally decreases as cardiorespiratory fitness increases. The average resting heart rate is usually between 60 to 70 beats per

minute. A well-conditioned endurance athlete such as a marathon runner can have a resting heart rate as low as 30 to 40 beats per minute. Conversely, a sedentary, unfit individual can have a resting heart rate of as much as 90 to 100 beats per minute.

4. Time of day: Resting heart rate increases throughout the day—it is lower in the morning and higher in the late afternoon and evening. This increase is influenced by the body's circadian rhythm (body clock) and the hormonal and biochemical changes that occur over 24 hours (see Question 15).

Four methods for determining heart rate training zones are available to athletes. Some methods are more reliable than others. The one that an athlete selects will depend on how serious an athlete is about his or her training and its monitoring. The four methods include the following:

1. VO_2 max testing (see Question 27): This is the single most accurate and reliable method of testing an athlete's heart rate responses to changing workloads. Unfortunately, this method may be out of reach (cost, availability) for most athletes.

2. 220 − age (age in years): This is a rough and ready formula that is used to determine the heart rate maximum. It is easy and convenient to use, but it has limitations. The major limitation is that it does not take into consideration the tremendous variability in an individual athlete's heart rates.

3. 208 − (0.7 × age) (age in years): This more recent equation takes into account the inevitable decline in heart rate with age.

4. Karvonen formula, training heart rate = (heart rate maximum − resting heart rate) × intensity + resting heart rate: Next to VO_2 max testing, the Karvonen

formula is probably the single best predictor of heart rate intensity. This method is often referred to as the heart rate reserve method, as it takes into account an athlete's resting heart rate. Earlier, it was mentioned that there was significant variability between individual athletes' resting heart rates. Athletes must establish an accurate resting heart rate by taking their pulse on awakening in the morning. The pulse should be taken over a 3-day period to ensure consistency; the average of the 3 days should then be calculated.

■ *Case Study*

Kelly is a 30-year-old runner who is preparing to run the Boston Marathon. She has been training regularly for 5 months and is getting close to the competition. Kelly wants to run the marathon at 70% of her heart rate maximum, and she is going to use all three formulas to see what provides her with the best results.

1. Heart rate maximum = 220 − age

    220 − 30 = 190 beats per minute

    70% of heart rate maximum = 190 × 0.7 (intensity)
    = 133 beats per minute

    Using this method, Kelly would want to compete at a constant HR of 133 beats per minute.

2. Heart rate maximum = 208 − (0.7 × age)

    208 − (0.7 × 30)

    208 − 21 = 187 beats per minute

    70% of heart rate maximum = 187 × 0.7
    = 130 beats per minute

    Using this more accurate formula, Kelly would want to compete at a constant heart rate of 130 beats per minute.

3. Karvonen formula: training heart rate = (heart rate maximum − resting heart rate) × intensity + resting heart rate

Kelly calculated her resting heart rate to be 50 beats per minute (this was calculated by taking an average 3-day heart rate first thing in the morning).

Heart rate maximum is calculated by using the 220 − age equation: 220 − 30 = 190 beats per minute.

Therefore, training heart rate = (heart rate maximum − resting heart rate) × intensity + resting heart rate

Training heart rate = (190 − 50) × 0.7 + 50

140 × 0.7 + 50 = 98 + 50 = 148 beats per minute

By comparing the various formulas for determining exercise heart rate at 70% intensity, there is evidently a significant disparity between the various methods: 133, 130, and 148 beats per minute. An athlete should experiment with each heart rate method to determine which formula is better suited for his or her level of intensity. If an athlete is familiar and confident in the use of the RPE scale (see Question 25), he or she should compare each heart rate outcome with a 12–13 (somewhat hard) for a reliable comparison. If one particular heart rate generates a 10–11 (fairly light) on the RPE scale, then an athlete should increase to the next higher heart rate.

An athlete should experiment with each heart rate method to determine which formula is better suited for his or her level of intensity.

Resting metabolic rate (RMR)

The minimum amount of energy required to meet the energy demands of the body while at rest. The resting metabolic rate is typically measured instead of BMR because it is only slightly higher than BMR and is determined under less rigorous conditions.

32. What is the resting metabolic rate? How is it measured? Why is it beneficial to know?

The **resting metabolic rate** (RMR) or **basal metabolic rate** is the amount of energy required to carry out the body's basic functions of respiration, circulation, and thermal regulation during a 24-hour period

Basal metabolic rate

The minimum amount of energy required to sustain life in the waking state. The basal metabolic rate is usually measured in the laboratory under very rigorous conditions.

while in a resting state. Several factors influence resting metabolic rate, including gender, height, weight, and percentage of lean muscle mass.

Resting metabolic rate can be a beneficial tool for an athlete in helping to regulate and maintain an ideal body weight. The resting metabolic rate ranges between 60% and 65% of an individual's total energy expenditure, and knowing it can be useful in helping athletes to achieve weight goals and optimize athletic performance. The resting metabolic rate is usually measured using a sophisticated, noninvasive breath analysis technique. The procedure takes approximately 30 minutes to complete and is designed to measure an individual's oxygen consumption to carbon dioxide output. The ratio of oxygen consumed to carbon dioxide produced in a relaxed, resting state will help to determine how much carbohydrate, fat, and total energy (calories) an individual is burning at rest.

To help ensure breath analysis accuracy, the clinician will try to control the following individual variables:

1. Avoid eating approximately 2 hours prior to testing.
2. Avoid exercise the day before and day of the test.
3. Avoid ingesting stimulant-based products such as caffeine, nicotine, or certain medications or supplements on test day, as these products have the potential to influence metabolic rate, thus resulting in inaccurate data.

Because it is not feasible for all athletes to get a resting metabolic rate test, it can also be estimated using a simple formula that requires an individual's weight, height, age, and activity level. Formulas are only estimates and can have error rates of between 100 and

200 calories per day compared with breath analysis techniques. One of the most accurate energy equations is the Mifflin St. Jeor:

Female: (10 × weight) + (6.25 × height) − (5 × age) − 161

Male: (10 × weight) + (6.25 × height) − (5 × age) + 5

Weight in kilograms (1 kilogram = 2.2 pounds)

Height in centimeters (1 inch = 2.54 centimeters)

Activity Factors:

1.200 = sedentary (little or no exercise)

1.375 = lightly active (light exercise/sports 1–3 days/ week)

1.550 = moderately active (moderate exercise/sports 3–5 days/week)

1.725 = very active (hard exercise/sports 6–7 days a week)

1.900 = extra active (very hard exercise/sports and physical job)

■ *Case Study* ————————————————

A 21-year-old, 6-foot (72 inch), 175-pound female collegiate basketball player wants to know her resting metabolic rate. She does not have access to the breath analysis technique but is advised to use the Mifflin St. Jeor equation as a reliable substitute.

Female: (10 × weight) + (6.25 × height) − (5 × age) − 161

Weight in kilograms (1 kilogram = 2.2 pounds) = 175/2.2 = 79.5 kilograms

Height in centimeters (1 inch = 2.54 centimeters)
= 72 × 2.54 = 182.9 centimeters

(10 × 79.5) + (6.25 × 182.9) − (5 × 21) − 161 = 1,672 calories per day without activity level factor

1,672 calories per day × 1.725 = 2,884 calories per day

1,672 calories per day × 1.900 = 3,176 calories per day

The recommend caloric intake for this athlete is 2,884 − 3,176 calories per day

33. What is the Wingate power test? Why is it important? How is it measured?

Wingate power test

The gold standard to assess muscle power, muscle endurance, and muscle fatigability.

The **Wingate power test** was developed during the 1970s at the Department of Research and Sports Medicine of the Wingate Institute for Physical Education and Sport in Israel. Since its introduction, the test has become the gold standard around the world for assessing muscle power, muscle endurance, and muscle fatigability. The test has been used as a reproducible standardized method to analyze physiological responses to high-intensity exercise. The Wingate power test is an excellent method to evaluate an athlete's peak power, mean (average) power, and muscle fatigability. A cyclist climbing a steep hill during a race, for example, would require maximal or near maximal force in order to be able to advance ahead of other competitors. Training for maximum power output, in this case, could make the difference between this cyclist being in the middle or at the head of the pack.

The Wingate power test for the lower torso is conducted on a stationary bike ergometer that measures power output in either watts or Newtons. After a thorough warm-up, the athlete is given the command "go," at which point the athlete cycles at maximum effort for the duration of 30 seconds. The highest 3 to 5 seconds of power output will be used to determine peak power, and the average 30-second power output will be used to determine mean power. Muscle fatigue can be graphed demonstrating percentage decreases in muscle power output over the 30 seconds. After 15 to 20 minutes of complete recovery, a second test may be administered, as needed. The exercise physiologist graphs the data to help identify strengths and potential deficiencies in the athlete's power output. This information can then be used by the exercise physiologist to help design a training program for improving the athlete's peak and mean power output while reducing muscle fatigability. A Wingate power test is also available for evaluating upper-torso power—particularly useful for athletes who participate in rowing, swimming, and boxing events.

34. What is the running economy test? How is it measured? Why is it important?

The **running economy test** is a laboratory assessment that is conducted by an experienced exercise physiologist to determine the efficiency of a runner's muscles, joints, and pulmonary system (lungs). The test requires an athlete to run on a treadmill set at a standard speed and elevation while attached to a metabolic cart that measures the amount of oxygen the athlete consumes at a pre-determined workload based on the athlete's body mass. The less oxygen an athlete requires during the test, the more efficient he or she is with his or her running and the less energy he or she will expend at that effort.

A running economy test is an excellent means of determining how much energy an athlete expends while exercising at a specific workload. Research has

Running economy test

A laboratory assessment to determine the efficiency of a runner's muscles, joints, and pulmonary system (lungs).

demonstrated that economical runners generally outperform less economical runners with similar physical and physiological attributes, as they tend to consume less oxygen for an identical amount of work. In other words, at a given speed of running, economical runners may not need to work as hard or use as much energy, which enables them to train and compete with greater intensity.

Running economy is measured on a treadmill. The athlete is attached to a metabolic cart and will run at a predetermined workload based on the athlete's body mass. The test is usually conducted in a laboratory setting by an experienced exercise physiologist. Running economy can vary between 1% and 4% from one day to the next and can be significantly improved with a well-designed exercise program involving strength development, sprinting, and overspeed training

■ *Case Study*

Sam, a marathon runner with 7 years of experience, has been sent by his coach to the performance laboratory for a running economy test. His coach believes that Sam is having difficulty with his running efficiency and believes that it can be improved. Sam's running economy test results confirmed that he does indeed have a slight deficit in his running efficiency. The exercise physiologist designed a 12-week sports-specific program that involved strength, sprint, and overspeed training. The second test, conducted 12 weeks later, revealed a 5% improvement in Sam's overall running economy. This improvement resulted in a 15-second per mile decrease in Sam's marathon time. His minute per mile pace improved from 6:25 minutes per mile pace to a 6:10-minute per mile pace, a significant improvement.

Before-, During-, and After- Exercise Nutrition

What should I eat before exercise?

Should I eat before an early-morning workout?

What types of foods should the athlete consume during exercise?

More ...

Before-exercise, during-exercise, and after-exercise, nutritional strategies are commonly ignored and poorly executed by athletes because of a fundamental lack of understanding and appreciation of performance benefits. Part Three builds on Part One by providing an athlete with specific nutritional strategies that are easy to implement with the ultimate benefit of providing an athlete with the performance edge.

35. What should I eat before exercise?

An athlete should consume a high-carbohydrate snack that is low in fat and protein about 30 to 60 minutes before practice or competition.

An athlete should consume a high-carbohydrate snack that is low in fat and protein about 30 to 60 minutes before practice or competition. The snack will provide energy and help to prevent hunger that may hinder performance. Foods that are high in carbohydrates will digest quickly and fuel the muscles for exercise. Avoid eating foods that are high in protein or fat, as they will take longer to digest and may cause stomach upset. Excellent pre-exercise snacks include fruit, granola bars, raisins, a bagel or English muffin with jelly, dry cereal, and high-carbohydrate energy bars.

Quick Fact

In contrast to popular belief, athletes should not exercise on an empty stomach assuming that it will burn more fat. There is no scientific evidence to substantiate this claim. There is evidence, however, that not consuming some type of food or fluid before exercise could decrease performance.

36. Should I eat before an early-morning workout?

An athlete should consume a high-carbohydrate snack that is low in protein and fat about 30 to 60 minutes before exercise. Some athletes find it hard to consume food early in the morning because of a suppressed appetite; however, the athlete should try to consume some type of carbohydrate before exercise. If he or she is unable to wake early enough to consume a snack (30 to 60 minutes before exercise), then an eating plan that provides the necessary fuel should be developed. Complaints of stomach upset are common when consuming foods too close to the start of exercise. This is usually avoidable by gradually building up from fluids to solid foods. The stomach should be trained, like muscles, with incremental increases in food/fluid and not by overloading too quickly. These gradual steps are designed to help the stomach adapt.

The following is a sample of an incremental morning snack plan. The athlete should follow a plan daily for 1 to 2 weeks to allow the stomach to adapt.

Week 1: 8-ounce sports drink (such as Gatorade, Powerade, Accelerade)

Week 2: 8-ounce fruit juice (apple, cranberry, and grape are recommended). Avoid orange and grapefruit juice, as they are highly acidic and may aggravate **acid reflux** and/or gastrointestinal distress.

Week 3: One-half banana or one-half granola bar

Week 4: Whole banana or whole granola bar

This plan is one possible menu out of many that an athlete may try. Athletes should experiment on their own with different foods and fluids to find what works best for them. Remember to select foods and fluids that are palatable and convenient, provide the right source of energy, supply sufficient energy, and do not cause stomach upset.

Acid reflux

An abnormal condition in which the valve between the stomach and the esophagus is not functioning properly; therefore, the acid from the stomach rises into the esophagus, causing a burning feeling.

37. What types of foods should the athlete consume during exercise?

If an athlete finds that he or she is low on energy during practice or competition, eating a high-carbohydrate snack that is low in fat and protein can be beneficial. The suggested carbohydrate intake during exercise is 30 to 60 grams per hour. It is often difficult to stop and eat while exercising; therefore, consuming convenient, prepackaged snacks such as raisins, Fig Newtons, energy gels, energy bars, sports beans, and sports drinks are highly recommended. These products provide a quick and easy way for the athlete to get the necessary energy back into his or her body during exercise and help to avoid the pitfall of premature fatigue.

Quick Fact

During ultra endurance events, athletes should consider adding a small amount of protein to their regular carbohydrate supplement in order to prevent excessive muscle breakdown and potential premature fatigue.

38. Why do I sometimes get a stomach upset after consuming energy gels or other concentrated forms of carbohydrates during exercise?

Stomach upsets are not uncommon among athletes who consume concentrated sources of carbohydrates during exercise. The stomach has the capacity to absorb approximately 1 liter (34 ounces) of fluid and 60 grams of carbohydrate per hour of exercise. Exceeding this amount can lead to gastrointestinal problems and impair performance. Carbohydrate sources

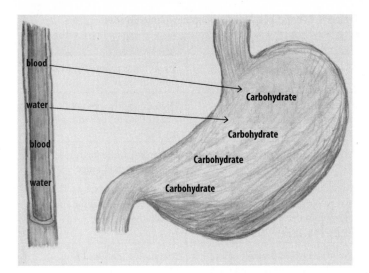

Figure 8   A high carbohydrate content in the stomach pulls water and blood into the stomach from the bloodstream. This can lead to bloating, cramps, and diarrhea.

concentrating in the stomach result in blood being pulled from the circulation (intestinal lumen) to aid the carbohydrate digestion (**Figure 8**). This stomach pooling can cause cramping, bloating, diarrhea, and vomiting. To avoid these problems, the athlete should consume plenty of water with the carbohydrates to assist in digestion and absorption (see Question 40).

39. What are the benefits of consuming water during exercise?

Water is one of the most important nutrients for athletic success. Water constitutes approximately 60% of the body's weight and should be maintained at that level for optimal performance. The importance of water is shown in **Table 9**.

Table 9   Benefits of Water Consumption During Exercise

Benefit	Mechanism
Maintains thermoregulation (cooling).	Sweat helps to remove heat from the body.
Preserves a high cardiac output, which reduces **cardiovascular strain**.	Water optimizes blood flow and oxygen to the working muscles.
Reduces **cardiac drift**, thus helping to reduce fatigue and premature "bonking".	Water keeps the heart rate within a normal range.
Keeps nutrients and oxygen flowing to the working muscle to prolong performance.	Oxygen is essential for energy production.
Increases waste product or metabolite removal to aid recovery.	Metabolites can lead to premature fatigue.
Reduces loss of mental focus and helps to increase **situational awareness**.	Water reduces injury and maintains a high level of performance.

Cardiovascular strain

Strain put on the cardiovascular system (heart and blood vessels).

Cardiac drift

An increase in heart rate as a result of decreased central blood volume caused by dehydration or blood loss.

Situational awareness

Aware of the surrounding environment within space and time.

Ambient temperature

Air temperature.

40. What types of fluids should I consume during exercise?

Adequate hydration is the key to a successful practice or competition. An athlete should consume approximately 5 to 12 ounces of fluid every 15 to 20 minutes during exercise. If exercise lasts less than 60 minutes, there is no need to consume sports drinks; water is adequate. If the athlete knows that the activity will last longer than 60 minutes or if the water (pool/open water) or **ambient temperature** is high, causing higher than normal sweat rates, sports drinks are proven to be beneficial and should be consumed from the start of exercise. The athlete should not wait until after the 60-minute period to begin consuming sports drinks. The athlete should follow the same drinking protocol for water—5 to 12 ounces of fluid every 15 to 20 minutes.

> **Quick Fact**
>
> 1 gulp of fluid = approximately 1 ounce

41. What factors influence an athlete's sweat loss during exercise?

Sweat is the primary means by which athletes lose heat from their body. Fluid loss, in the form of sweat, is dependent on several factors, including **body surface area**, external environmental temperature, genetics, heat acclimatization, initial hydration status, type of clothing worn, and intensity/duration of exercise (**Table 10**). An athlete must be aware that respiratory and **urinary losses** can also compound dehydration. Athletes sweat in both warm and cool environments,

Body surface area

Calculation or measurement of the body's surface.

Urinary losses

Loss of macronutrients and micronutrients via urination.

Before-, During-, and After-Exercise Nutrition

Table 10 Factors That Influence Sweat Rates and Their Impact on Athletes

Factors	Impact
Body surface area.	A larger athlete will lose more fluids through sweating than a smaller athlete.
External environmental temperature.	Higher temperatures will result in higher sweat rates.
Genetics.	Sweat rates are inherited.
Heat acclimatization.	A well-conditioned and acclimated athlete sweats more, sweats faster, and loses more sodium than an unconditioned and unacclimated athlete; therefore, fluid and sodium needs are higher for the acclimated athlete.
Initial hydration status.	A hydrated athlete will sweat more than a dehydrated athlete.
Type of clothing worn.	In warm weather, select clothing that is light in color, lightweight, and breathable (aerated) to prevent overheating. In cold weather, select clothing that is lightweight, warm, and capable of wicking moisture away from the skin's surface to prevent chilling.
Intensity/duration of exercise.	The harder and longer the exercise, the more the athlete sweats.

and each athlete must be attentive to his or her own body's sweat response to exercise.

42. What should I eat after exercise to maximize my recovery?

Thirty minutes after a workout, an athlete should consume a high-carbohydrate snack with a small amount of protein. This strategy has proven to be very effective for those athletes working out more than one time per day several days per week or after intense training sessions that last 30 minutes or longer. The first 30 minutes is the optimal time for the athlete to begin restoring the glycogen lost during exercise and commence the process of rebuilding muscle tissue. Glycogen stores take approximately 20 to 22 hours to replenish fully as long as the athlete is consuming the recommended amounts of carbohydrate and eating consistently throughout the rest of the day. Missing a post-workout snack may result in premature muscle fatigue and prolonged soreness caused by incomplete glycogen restoration. **Figure 9** represents muscle glycogen depletion caused by successive days of intensive exercise without adequate carbohydrate consumption. Not eating after exercise could negatively affect the athlete's next practice or competition and may increase the likelihood of injury.

Glycogen stores take approximately 20 to 22 hours to replenish fully as long as the athlete is consuming the recommended amounts of carbohydrate and eating consistently throughout the rest of the day.

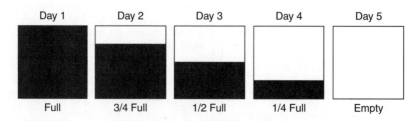

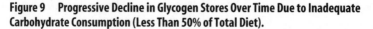

Figure 9   Progressive Decline in Glycogen Stores Over Time Due to Inadequate Carbohydrate Consumption (Less Than 50% of Total Diet).

Research has demonstrated that glycogen restoration within the first 2 hours after exercise is approximately 8% per hour when consuming carbohydrate alone. After this 2-hour period, the glycogen restoration rate drops to approximately 5% per hour. Adding a small amount of protein with the carbohydrate within the first 2 hours after exercise has been shown to increase **glycogen synthesis** to as much as 10% (2% more than consuming carbohydrates alone).

Excellent post-workout snacks include a peanut butter and jelly sandwich, chocolate milk or other flavored milks, smoothies, low-fat yogurt, trail mix, cereal with milk, fruit, and energy bars. Some athletes complain of a low appetite after workout and do not want to consume solids foods. In these cases, liquid foods such as smoothies and flavored milks are appropriate.

Glycogen synthesis
A biological process for increasing the amount of glycogen in the liver and muscle cells.

■ *Case Study* ────────────────────

Iezzy, a 16-year-old gymnast, complains of soreness, fatigue, and heavy legs for several days after a hard practice. Practices start at 5 p.m. and usually last for 3 to 4 hours during the week, and on the weekends practice lasts 5 to 6 hours. Iezzy tells the sports dietitian that on most days during the week (not on the weekends) she skips eating after workouts because she needs to finish her homework and go to bed. The sports dietitian explains to Iezzy that the heaviness felt in her legs, fatigue, and soreness are most likely related to the lack of glycogen in her system. After workouts, Iezzy must consume a snack that is high in carbohydrates and low in proteins and fats within 30 minutes to immediately begin restoring the glycogen lost and to rebuild muscle tissue. Iezzy needs to implement these two items into her busy daily schedule: (1) a snack while in the car going to and from practice and (2) liquids, such as smoothies, chocolate milk, or other flavored milks, while she is studying. Within a few days of consuming a snack immediately after each practice, Iezzy reported that her symptoms disappeared, allowing her to perform better in the gym and in the classroom.

43. What types of carbohydrates are recommended to restore muscle glycogen immediately (within 30 minutes) after exercise?

Sucrose

A commonly consumed sugar also known as table sugar. It is composed of glucose and fructose.

Fructose

A simple sugar, commonly found in fruits, that is known for its sweet taste.

Simple carbohydrates in the form of glucose and **sucrose** should be immediately consumed after exercise. Simple carbohydrates are rapidly digested and absorbed from the stomach into the circulation, stimulating faster recovery of the athlete's glycogen stores. Some good sources include flavored milks, sports drinks, and energy gels. Using concentrated forms of **fructose** (citrus juices) as the sole source of post-exercise energy replacement should be avoided, as they take longer to be digested and can cause gastrointestinal distress, including cramping, diarrhea (electrolyte losses and dehydration), and bloating. Complex starches should also be avoided after exercise, as they take longer to digest and be absorbed into the circulation, possibly delaying recovery.

> ## Quick Fact
> White bread instead of wheat bread is recommended after a workout to ensure rapid digestion and absorption.

The suggested amount of simple carbohydrates consumed after exercise is 1.5 grams per kilogram of body weight in the first 30 minutes and then an additional 1.5 grams per kilogram every 2 hours thereafter, which can be consumed as complex starches.

44. What source of protein should I consume after exercise, whey or casein?

The two most common forms of protein that athletes prefer to consume include whey and casein. Whey protein is a biproduct of cheese manufacturing. It is a short **peptide-bonded protein** and is rapidly digested and absorbed into the circulation (bloodstream). **Caseinated protein**, on the other hand, has a longer peptide-bonded structure and is digested at a slower rate. Whey protein is found in yogurt and cottage cheese (the liquid on the surface of the product before it is mixed), and caseinated protein is found in milk. After exercise, whey protein has been shown to be more effective for the athlete to consume, as it is digested and absorbed into the circulation faster than caseinated protein. The quicker absorption of whey protein may enable athletes to begin their muscle recovery sooner. Whey protein has been widely researched and proven to be the most effective protein source for increasing lean body mass, strength, power, and **work capacity**, and for decreasing fat mass. The recommended amount of protein necessary to attain the previously mentioned benefits is no more than 1.5 grams per kilogram of body weight per day; athletes who consume more than the recommended amounts will *not* incur any additional gains and could have poorer performance.

Certain athletes may have an adverse reaction to the consumption of whey protein. Whey protein is a dairy biproduct, and athletes who are lactose intolerant may experience symptoms that are similar to those that are felt after milk ingestion. For lactose-intolerant individuals, **soy protein** has proven to be an effective alternative to whey/caseinated protein.

Peptide-bonded protein

A molecular chain compound composed of two or more amino acids joined by peptide bonds.

Caseinated protein

Long peptide-bonded structure that is digested at a slower rate than whey protein. Caseinated protein is found in milk.

Work capacity

The capacity to do work.

Soy protein

A protein source made from soybeans.

Protein should come from a variety of food sources in the athlete's daily diet, not solely from supplementation through the use of powders and liquids.

45. What is the optimal amount of carbohydrates and protein that should be consumed after a workout or competition?

In order for an athlete to maximize his or her post-workout recovery, the right combination of carbohydrate and protein must be consumed. The type of sport or activity will determine what ratio of carbohydrate to protein should be consumed. When glycogen stores are depleted, an athlete should ingest sufficient quantities of carbohydrate and protein to restore glycogen adequately and enhance muscle repair. The recommended goal is to consume these foods within 30 minutes after exercise. This 30-minute window is essential to enhancing recovery. The guidelines in **Table 11** provide the proper amounts of nutrients needed to optimize recovery for endurance and strength athletes. The carbohydrate to protein ratio will vary between endurance and strength athletes because the mode and goal of the exercise differs. These recommendations do not need to be followed if there will be more than one to two days between intense training sessions.

46. What is the purpose of carbohydrate loading?

Supercompensate

A method that increases glycogen stores beyond the cell's normal capacity.

Cellular glycogen

Amount of glycogen stored in the cells.

Carbohydrate loading (carbo-loading) is a highly effective method that athletes use to **supercompensate** their **cellular glycogen** stores approximately 72 hours before competition. Carbo-loading is accomplished by increasing carbohydrate consumption to as much as 70% to 80% of total caloric intake and simultaneously decreasing exercise duration and intensity (**tapering**).

Table 11   Immediate and Long-Term Post-Workout Carbohydrate and Protein Requirements for Endurance and Strength Athletes

Endurance Athletes	Strength Athletes
3 to 4 grams carbohydrate:1 gram of protein 30 to 40 grams of carbohydrate and 8 to 10 grams of protein	2 grams carbohydrate:1 gram protein 30 to 40 grams of carbohydrate and 15 to 20 grams of protein
Carbohydrate intake: 1.5 grams per kilogram of body weight during the first 30 minutes and then 1.5 grams per kilogram every 2 hours for 4 to 6 hours after workout	Carbohydrate intake: 1.5 grams per kilogram of body weight during the first 30 minutes and then 1.5 grams per kilogram every 2 hours for 4 to 6 hours after workout
Sources: chocolate milk (or other flavored milks), cereal with skim or 1% milk, fruit with peanut butter, energy bar with the above amount of carbohydrate:protein	Sources: one-third cup of trail mix, one-half cup peanut butter or a 2-ounce turkey sandwich, one-half cup cereal with skim or 1% milk, energy bar with the above amount of carbohydrate:protein
Example: a triathlete weighing 175 pounds (79.5 kilograms, 1 kilogram = 2.2 pounds) post-exercise nutritional requirements are: carbohydrates: 79.5 kilograms × 1.5 gram per kilogram = 119 grams protein: = 39 grams (4:1 ratio of carbohydrate:protein)	Example: a power lifter weighing 175 pounds (79.5 kilograms, 1 kilogram = 2.2 pounds) post-exercise nutritional requirements are: carbohydrates: 79.5 kilograms × 1.5 grams per kilogram = 119 grams protein: = 78 grams (2:1 ratio of carbohydrate:protein)

Glycogen stores can be doubled above normal levels, which may prolong endurance performance by as much as 60 minutes or more. Carbo-loading is most beneficial to athletes who are engaged in exercise lasting 90 minutes or longer. Some athletes who have carbo-loaded have commented that the method has produced a sense of fullness or heaviness in their limbs. This can be attributed to the fact that for every gram of glycogen stored in the muscle cell there is approximately 3 grams of water stored along with it. To date, there is no evidence that this feeling of fullness or heaviness adversely affects the athlete's performance.

Tapering

A scheduled decrease in the volume and intensity of training six or more days prior to competition. The purpose is to allow for recovery from training and replenishment of glycogen stores in the liver and muscle.

Before-, During-, and After-Exercise Nutrition

87

> **Quick Fact**
>
> Two hours of endurance exercise at 70% VO_2 max can significantly drain muscle and liver glycogen stores.

47. How do I carbo-load?

Carbo-loading is usually begun six days before competition.

Carbo-loading is usually begun six days before competition. For the first three days, the athlete will reduce his or her training intensity (≤50% of VO_2 max) while maintaining normal training volume and eating his or her usual mixed diet. For the three days before competition, the athlete will reduce training volume to a duration of no more than 15 minutes of very light exercise similar to that of a warm-up while increasing his or her dietary carbohydrate consumption to no less than 70% of his or her total calorie intake. **Figure 10** shows the inverse relationship between exercise intensity and duration with carbohydrate consumption.

Glycemic index

An index for classifying carbohydrate foods based on how quickly they are digested and absorbed into the bloodstream. The more quickly blood glucose rises after ingestion, the higher the glycemic index.

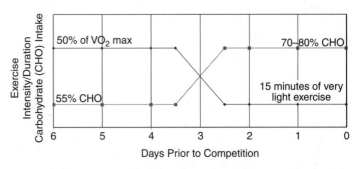

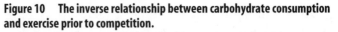

Figure 10   The inverse relationship between carbohydrate consumption and exercise prior to competition.

Blood glucose response

Measurement of how circulating blood glucose responds to an increase or a decrease in food intake.

48. What is the glycemic index, and how can it be used to improve my performance?

The **glycemic index** is a ranking of carbohydrate foods based on their measured **blood glucose response** compared with a food reference, either glucose or white bread. Blood glucose responds, or rises, after the ingestion of carbohydrate. The rate at which it rises is based on how rapidly it is digested and absorbed into the bloodstream; the faster it is digested, the higher the food ranks on the glycemic index scale. **Table 12** provides a list of common foods and their glycemic index rankings.

Table 12   Glycemic Index and Glycemic Load of Common Foods

Food	Glycemic Index (Glucose = 100)	Glycemic Index (White Bread = 100)	Glycemic Index Category*	Serving Size (g)	g CHO/ serving	Glycemic Load
White bread, Wonder	73 ± 2	105 ± 3	High	30	14	10
White rice, boiled	64 ± 7	91 ± 9	High	150	36	23
Couscous	65 ± 4	93 ± 6	High	150	35	23
Gatorade	78 ± 13	111	High	250 mL	5	12
Ice cream	61 ± 7	87 ± 10	High	50	13	8
Sweet potato	61 ± 7	87 ± 10	High	150	28	17
Baked potato, russet	85 ± 12	121 ± 16	High	150	30	26
Cranberry juice cocktail	68 ± 3	97	High	250 mL	6	24
Grapenuts	71 ± 4	102 ± 6	High	30	21	15
Cornflakes	81 ± 3	116 ± 5	High	30	26	21
Blueberry muffin	59	84 ± 8	High	57	29	17
Power bar	56 ± 3	79 ± 4	Med	65	42	24
Honey	55 ± 5	78 ± 7	Med	25	18	10
White rice, long grain	56 ± 2	80 ± 3	Med	150	41	23
Coca-Cola	58 ± 5	83 ± 7	Med	250 mL	6	16

Table 12   Glycemic Index and Glycemic Load of Common Foods (*Continued*)

Food	Glycemic Index (Glucose = 100)	Glycemic Index (White Bread = 100)	Glycemic Index Category*	Serving Size (g)	g CHO/ˋ serving	Glycemic Load
Sweet corn	54 ± 4	78 ± 6	Med	80	17	9
Carrot	47 ± 16	68 ± 23	Med	80	6	3
New potato	57 ± 7	81 ± 10	Med	150	21	12
Banana	52 ± 4	74 ± 5	Med	120	24	12
Orange juice	50 ± 4	71 ± 5	Med	250 mL	26	13
Chickpeas	28 ± 6	39 ± 8	Low	150	30	8
Kidney beans	28 ± 4	39 ± 6	Low	150	25	7
Xylitol	8 ± 1	11 ± 1	Low	10	10	1
Lentils	29 ± 1	41 ± 1	Low	150	18	5
Chocolate cake, frosted	38 ± 3	54	Low	111	52	20
Fructose	19 ± 2	27 ± 4	Low	10	10	2
Tomato juice	38 ± 4	54	Low	250 mL	9	4
Skim milk	32 ± 5	46	Low	250 mL	13	4
Smoothie, raspberry	33 ± 9	48 ± 13	Low	250 mL	41	14
Apple	38 ± 2	52 ± 3	Low	120	15	6

* Category = High (> 85); Medium (60–85); Low (< 60) using GI white bread = 100

Source: Adapted from Foster-Powell K, Holt SHA, Brand-Miller JC. International table of glycemic index and glycemic load values. *Am J Clin Nutr* 2002;76:5–56.

The glycemic index can be a valuable tool for athletes to use as part of their sports nutrition plan; however, an athlete must be aware of its potential disadvantages. Research has demonstrated that high-, medium-, and low-glycemic index foods play specific roles before, during, and after exercise. **Table 13** provides recommendations on how to use the glycemic index.

Table 13   Before-, During-, and After-Workout Glycemic Index Recommendations

When?	What?	Why?
Before workout	Low-to-medium glycemic index foods	• Minimize potential spikes in blood sugar (reactive hypoglycemia), which can occur at the beginning of exercise in some athletes and may cause a sense of sluggishness • Increasing amounts of circulating fats in the blood, possibly providing more energy for exercise • Increase fat utilization, reducing reliance on carbohydrate as fuel (glycogen sparing) • May enhance endurance performance
During workout	Medium-to-high glycemic index foods	• Provides muscles a quick delivery of carbohydrate energy to optimize performance • Avoid low-glycemic-index foods, as they may decrease performance and cause gastrointestinal distress
After workout	Medium-to-high glycemic index foods	• Helps replenish glycogen stores immediately after exercise, enhancing recovery

The glycemic index does have some disadvantages if used as the exclusive method for nutrition preparation. The ranking of foods on the glycemic index scale can be influenced by one or more of the following:

1. The type and amount of carbohydrate being consumed vary.

2. Different soils can produce identical foods that vary in glycemic index values.

3. Soluble versus insoluble fiber can affect digestion rates.

4. Foods high in protein and fat empty from the stomach at a slower rate than carbohydrates. Because

humans normally consume a mixed diet of carbohydrates, fats, and proteins, glycemic index levels may vary because of the slower rate at which glucose enters the circulation (versus a single food source).

5. Liquids are generally digested and absorbed at a faster rate than solids.

6. Undigested foods from a previous meal or snack may reduce the rate of digestion and absorption of the next feeding.

7. The time of day can influence the rate at which carbohydrates are digested and absorbed because of fluctuations in gut motility and digestive enzyme production.

Athletes who fully comprehend the concepts of the glycemic index will be able to incorporate some beneficial strategies into their nutritional plan, optimizing their performance and recovery.

Vitamins and Minerals

What role do vitamins play in an athlete's diet?

What role do minerals play in an athlete's diet?

What role does calcium play in athletic performance?

More . . .

Part Four details the importance of vitamins and minerals for good health and athletic performance. This section identifies some the more common deficiencies that athletes may experience and provides a detailed explanation on causes, effects, and prevention. By ignoring this information, an athlete may risk jeopardizing his or her health and performance.

49. What role do vitamins play in an athlete's diet?

Vitamins play an important role in the bodily functions that are necessary for good health and performance. Vitamins are classified as either water soluble or fat soluble. **Water-soluble vitamins** dissolve in water and are easily transported in the blood. They include vitamin C, choline, and the B complex vitamins (thiamin, riboflavin, niacin, B_6, B_{12}, folate, biotin, and pantothenic acid). Daily intake of water-soluble vitamins is necessary because they dissolve easily in water and cannot be stored in large amounts in the body. Excessive consumption of water-soluble vitamins will be excreted through urine. Water-soluble vitamins must be consumed on a daily basis in order to meet the Recommended Dietary Intake. **Fat-soluble vitamins** do not dissolve easily in water and require dietary fat for intestinal absorption and transport into the bloodstream. The fat-soluble vitamins are A, D, E, and K, and unlike many water-soluble vitamins, they can be stored in the body. Because fat-soluble vitamins are stored in higher quantities than water-soluble vitamins, the potential for fat-soluble vitamin toxicity exists. Vitamins play a significant role in the body, including energy production, hemoglobin synthesis, maintenance of bone health, immune function, protection of body tissues from oxidative damage, and building and repair of muscles after exercise. The functions

Water-soluble vitamins

A class of vitamins that dissolve in water and are easily transported in the blood. The water-soluble vitamins are the B vitamins, vitamin C, and choline.

Daily intake of water-soluble vitamins is necessary because they dissolve easily in water and cannot be stored in large amounts in the body.

Fat-soluble vitamins

A group of vitamins that does not dissolve easily in water and requires dietary fat for intestinal absorption and transport into the bloodstream. The fat soluble vitamins are A, D, E, and K.

and sources of water- and fat-soluble vitamins can be found in **Table 14**.

Exercise can increase the need for certain vitamins and minerals in athletes who engage in high-intensity and long-duration activities. These increases are likely related to higher sweat, urine, and feces losses and elevated production of **free radicals**. The amount of vitamins and minerals needed above the Recommended Dietary Intake or Adequate Intake (AI) are still being researched; therefore, it is important that athletes get yearly physicals to ensure that they are getting the proper amount of nutrients. Athletes should focus on attaining their vitamin and mineral needs from food sources as opposed to supplements, as the vitamins and minerals in foods are more **bioavailable**. The indiscriminate use of supplements over food by an athlete can increase the potential for toxicity (supplement overdose).

Free radicals

Highly reactive molecules, usually containing oxygen, that have unpaired electrons in their outer shell. Because of their highly reactive nature, free radicals have been implicated as culprits in diseases ranging from cancer to cardiovascular disease.

Bioavailable

The amount of an ingested nutrient that is absorbed and available to the body.

Vitamins and Minerals

Table 14   Functions and Sources of Water- and Fat-Soluble Vitamins

Vitamin	Water or Fat Soluble	Major Function	Signs of Deficiency	Sources
C	Water	Aids in collagen formation, wound healing, immune function, and maintaining blood vessels, bones, teeth	Wounds heal slowly, bleeding gums, dry skin, increased susceptibility to illness	Potatoes, broccoli, citrus fruits, melon, strawberries, tomatoes, green peppers, dark green vegetables, fortified juices
B₁ (thiamin)	Water	Is vital for nervous system function, releases energy from foods, promotes natural appetite and digestion	Impaired growth, mental confusion, edema, muscle weakness	Whole and enriched grain products, peas, meat, pork, legumes, liver, soybeans

(*Continued*)

95

Table 14   Functions and Sources of Water- and Fat-Soluble Vitamins (*Continued*)

Vitamin	Water or Fat Soluble	Major Function	Signs of Deficiency	Sources
B$_2$ (riboflavin)	Water	Supports good vision and healthy skin, helps release energy from foods, maintains integrity of skin, tongue, lips	Sensitivity to light (eyes), itchy skin, cracks at the corners of the mouth	Whole and enriched grain products, eggs, dark green vegetables, milk, liver
B$_6$ (pyridoxine)	Water	Aids in protein metabolism, helps red blood cell formation, aids the body in using fats	Skin disorders, anemia, cracks at the corners of the mouth, kidney stones, nausea	Whole grains and cereals, legumes, green leafy vegetables, meats, pork
B$_{12}$ (cyanocobal-amin)	Water	Helps build genetic material, maintain nervous system, development of red blood cells	Anemia, neurological disorders, degeneration of peripheral nerves that leads to numbness and tingling in fingers and toes	Only found in animal foods: meats, liver, eggs, milk, milk products, fish, oysters, shellfish, kidney
Niacin	Water	Aids in energy production from foods, promotes natural appetite, supports healthy skin and nerves, aids digestion	Mental confusion, skin disorders, irritability, weakness, diarrhea	Peanuts, poultry, meats, liver, fish, whole and enriched grain products
Biotin	Water	Aids in releasing energy from carbohydrates and fat synthesis	Fatigue, loss of appetite, anemia, muscle pains, nausea, depression	Egg yolk, milk, liver, kidney, salmon, fresh vegetables, soybeans, made by intestinal bacteria
Pantothenic acid	Water	Aids in formation of hormones, essential in energy production	Uncommon	Egg yolk, liver, kidney, legumes, whole grains, made by intestinal bacteria

Table 14   Functions and Sources of Water- and Fat-Soluble Vitamins (*Continued*)

Folic acid (folacin)	Water	Promotes red blood cell, prevents birth defects of the brain and spine, aids in protein metabolism, lowers homocysteine levels, therefore reducing risk of coronary artery disease	Anemia, gastrointestinal disturbances, smooth tongue	Whole grains, fortified cereals and grains, legumes, citrus fruits, green leafy vegetables, meats, fish, liver, kidney
Choline	Water	Aids in nervous system function and fat metabolism	Uncommon	Whole grains, legumes, milk, egg yolk, liver, meats
A (retinol)	Fat	Forms and keeps healthy skin and mucous membranes to increase resistance to infections, necessary for night vision and tooth and bone development	Night blindness, intestinal infections, diarrhea, keratinization of the skin and eyes	Vitamin A-fortified milk and dairy products, whole milk, cheese, egg yolk, liver, carrots, leafy green vegetables, sweet potatoes, pumpkins, winter squash, cantaloupe, apricots
D (calciferol)	Fat	Increases calcium absorption, supports hardening of the teeth and bones	Osteomalacia, rickets, delayed dentition	Vitamin D-fortified dairy products, fish oils, margarines, egg yolk, synthesized by the sun on the skin
E (alpha-tocopherol)	Fat	Prevents cell damage, antioxidant, protects vitamins A and C and fatty acids	Increase hemolysis of red blood cells in vitro, anemia and dermatitis in infants	Green and leafy vegetables, wheat germ, whole grain products, nuts, egg yolks, liver, vegetable oil, butter, margarine, shortening
K	Fat	Clots blood	Excessive bleeding, liver injury	Dark leafy greens, liver, made by bacteria in the intestine

Vitamins and Minerals

Quick Fact

Overcooking or inappropriately storing foods that contain high amounts of water-soluble vitamins can destroy and/or reduce the amount of vitamins available in the food. Produce should not be overcooked and should be refrigerated as soon as possible; milk and grains should not be kept in direct light for long periods of time, as direct sunlight can alter the nutritional value of the product and can adversely affect flavor.

Major minerals

The minerals required by the body in amounts greater than 100 milligrams per day. The major minerals include calcium, phosphorus, magnesium, sodium, chloride, potassium, and sulfur.

Trace minerals

Minerals required by the body in quantities less than 100 milligrams per day. The trace minerals include iron, zinc, chromium, fluoride, copper, manganese, iodine, molybdenum, and selenium.

Micronutrients

Essential nutrients (i.e., vitamins and trace minerals) required in only small quantities (milligrams and micrograms) by the body.

50. What role do minerals play in an athlete's diet?

Minerals are classified into two categories: major minerals and trace minerals. **Major minerals** are required by the body in amounts greater than 100 milligrams per day and include calcium, phosphorus, magnesium, sodium, chloride, potassium, and sulfur. **Trace minerals** are required by the body in amounts less than 100 milligrams per day and include iron, zinc, chromium, fluoride, copper, manganese, iodine, molybdenum, and selenium. The function and sources of major and trace minerals are found in **Table 15**.

Because exercise places specific stress on the metabolic pathways, an athlete's micronutrient requirements may need to be increased. High levels of training result in numerous muscle biochemical adaptations that increase the need for certain **micronutrients**. Athletes should focus on attaining their vitamins and minerals from food sources, as opposed to supplements, as vitamins and minerals in foods are more bioavailable. The indiscriminate use of supplements over food by an athlete can increase the potential for toxicity (supplement overdose).

Table 15   Function and Sources of Major and Trace Minerals

Mineral	Major or Trace Mineral	Major Function	Sources
Calcium	Major	Needed for strong bones and teeth, muscle contraction, blood clotting, energy production, keep immune system strong	Milk and other dairy products, green leafy vegetables, broccoli, salmon, sardines
Magnesium	Major	Essential for biological processes, activate enzymes involved in protein synthesis	Fish, nuts, beans, whole grains, green leafy vegetables, soybeans, wheat germ
Phosphorus	Major	Cell functions and membranes, strong bones and teeth	Fish, meats, eggs, poultry, vegetables, dairy products, nuts, cereals, whole grains
Potassium	Major	Muscle contraction, nerve conduction, energy production	Fresh fruits and vegetables
Sodium	Major	Water balance	Table salt, added to foods by food manufacturers
Chlorine	Major	Helps maintain the body's fluid and electrolyte balances, digestive juices	Table salt
Sulfur	Major	Sulfur-containing amino acids	Garlic, onions, dairy products, meat, eggs
Iron	Trace	Enzyme action for energy production, hemoglobin synthesis and function, collagen and elastin production	Poultry, fish, meat, organ meats, fortified grains and cereals
Zinc	Trace	Eyesight, immunity, and wound healing	Whole grains, fish, meat, brewer's yeast, pork, peanuts
Chromium	Trace	Uses sugar in the body	Whole grains, meat, brewer's yeast, black pepper
Copper	Trace	Synthesis and function of hemoglobin, collagen and elastin production, melanin formation	Nuts, fruits, shellfish, organ meats

(*Continued*)

Table 15   Function and Sources of Major and Trace Minerals (*Continued*)

Mineral	Major or Trace Mineral	Major Function	Sources
Fluorine	Trace	Binds calcium in teeth and bones	Fluoridated water, seafood, tea
Iodine	Trace	Energy production (part of thyroid hormones)	Iodized salt, seafood
Selenium	Trace	Constituent for numerous enzymes	Whole grains, onions, broccoli, cabbage, seafood, organ meats, celery, brewer's yeast
Manganese	Trace	Constituent for numerous enzymes	Nuts, whole grains, egg yolk, tea, green vegetables
Molybdenum	Trace	Constituent for numerous enzymes	Beans, milk, whole grains, green leafy vegetables, organ meats

Quick Fact

Athletes wanting to supplement and who do not have a micronutrient deficiency should look for a multivitamin source that does *not* exceed 100% of the Recommended Dietary Intake for any one particular vitamin or mineral.

51. What role does calcium play in athletic performance?

Calcium is one of the seven major minerals that the body needs; others include phosphorus, magnesium, sodium, chloride, potassium, and sulfur.

Calcium is one of the seven major minerals that the body needs; others include phosphorus, magnesium, sodium, chloride, potassium, and sulfur. Calcium plays a significant role in the body, as it is necessary for building and repairing bone and tooth tissue, maintaining blood calcium levels, clotting blood, and aiding in nerve function; it is also essential for muscle contraction, disease prevention, and even weight management.

Calcium intake has a positive impact on health and disease prevention. Research has found that foods rich in calcium are important in the prevention of osteoporosis, and they can reduce cardiovascular disease, decrease the incidence of colon cancer, and assist in weight management.

1. **Osteoporosis** means "porous bone" and usually affects older adults. This disease is characterized by decreased bone mineralization and is usually a product of poor bone formation during puberty. Osteoporosis weakens the bones and can result in an increased susceptibility to fractures. Osteoporosis is a preventable disease; consuming adequate calcium during maturation will help to decrease the likelihood of the disorder later in life. Calcium supplementation, along with weight bearing exercise, has been successfully used in helping to prevent and treat osteoporosis.

2. Cardiovascular disease is a condition that is characterized by reduced blood flow resulting from plaque build-up in the arteries of the heart. The blockage can lead to decreased blood flow and oxygen to the heart muscle, resulting in a heart attack and decreased blood flow to the brain leading to stroke. Research has shown that low-fat milk, non-fat milk, and other milk products (that contain calcium) have been linked to a decline in cardiovascular risk factors such as a decrease in low-density lipoprotein cholesterol, hypertension, and homocysteine levels and an improved total cholesterol profile.

3. Colon cancer is a disease that affects the **colon** and its ability to function properly. Cancer is an abnormal growth of cells throughout the colon. Recent research has concluded that the consumption of milk and milk products can significantly decrease the proliferation of colonic epithelial cells (slowing the rate of cancer cell growth), thus reducing one's susceptibility to the disease.

Osteoporosis
Means "porous bone" and usually affects older adults. This disease is characterized by decreased bone mineralization and is a product of poor bone formation during puberty. This disease weakens the bones and results in an increased susceptibility to fractures.

Colon
Part of the digestive system whose main function is to extract salt, water, and certain vitamins before they are eliminated from the body.

Vitamins and Minerals

Pandemic

An epidemic of a disease that is spreading through human populations across a large region such as a continent or several continents (worldwide).

4. Obesity is **pandemic** and is becoming an increasing healthcare concern for countries throughout the world. Many of the developed countries of the world are experiencing levels of overweight and obesity of 50% or more. As a result of this increased rate of obesity, healthcare costs to treat comorbidities (hypertension, diabetes, high cholesterol) associated with weight gain are escalating. Several controlled clinical studies on overweight and obese adults after reduced-calories diets containing dairy and calcium intake showed greater weight loss than those who followed a calorie-reduced diet only. Although not fully understood, it appears that the use of low-fat milk and milk products (with calcium) may help to regulate weight and body fat. Dairy products appear to have a pronounced effect on individual energy expenditure, fat burning, fat absorption, and satiety.

Quick Fact

Calcium is essential for bone growth and development. Peak bone mineralization is reached during puberty and adolescence. Peak bone mass is about 90% complete by 20 years of age. During this period, it is critical to consume foods that are high in calcium.

Calcium deficiency is relatively common in many athletes because of low calcium ingestion. Numerous young athletes, during their critical bone development, are reducing their calcium intake by replacing milk with higher levels of soda consumption. Recent studies have shown that high levels of phosphorus in commercial sodas can lead to the leaching of calcium from the bones. Soda consumption should be kept to a minimum and should not take the place of milk in the diet (see **Table 16** for calcium recommendations). One of the

Table 16   Adequate Intake for Calcium

Age (Years)	Calcium (Milligrams)
14–18	1,300
19–30	1,000
31–50	1,200
> 50	1,200
Females that are amenorrheic or those athletes with high sweat rates are recommended to consume higher amounts of calcium.	1,500–2,000

most common symptoms of calcium deficiency in athletes is muscle cramps. Muscle cramps, however, are not the best indicator of calcium deficiency because the body works to prevent cramps by pulling calcium from the bones. This insidious compensation can negatively affect bone health, leading to early-onset osteoporosis.

Calcium toxicity, consuming more than 2,500 milligrams per day, is typically the result of athletes consuming higher than normal amounts of calcium from supplements. Rarely is calcium toxicity seen by overconsumption of calcium-rich foods only. High calcium intakes lead to impaired absorption of other minerals (such as iron and zinc) and potentially to kidney stones; it may even lead to cardiac arrest caused by dysrhythmia.

Vitamin D plays an important role in the absorption and utilization of calcium. Vitamin D is a fat-soluble vitamin, and its main function is to control calcium levels in the blood regulating bone growth and development. Vitamin D synthesis is best accomplished through skin exposure to the sun, but frequent sun exposure is not always feasible or safe and should not be the athlete's sole source of vitamin D. Excessive sun contact may lead to increased susceptibility to skin cancer, and athletes competing in hot conditions where they may be exposed to large amounts of direct sunlight should use an effective sunscreen. Because most foods are naturally low in vitamin D, milk and cereals have been fortified with vitamin D to prevent health ramifications (such as osteoporosis).

Eating calcium-rich foods (see **Figure 11**) is recommended before taking a supplement. Some athletes, however, require supplements, as they simply do not enjoy foods that are rich in calcium or may be lactose

CALCIUM

Daily Value = 1000 mg
RDA = 1000 mg (males/females)

High: 20% DV or more	Food	Amount	Calcium
	Tofu, calcium processed	85 g (~1/3 cup)	581 mg
	Yogurt, plain, lowfat	225 g (1 8-oz container)	448 mg
	Milk, nonfat	240 ml (1 cup)	352 mg
	Milk, 2% milkfat	240 ml (1 cup)	352 mg
	Milk, 1% milkfat	240 ml (1 cup)	349 mg
	Sesame seeds, whole roasted, toasted	30 g (~1 oz)	297 mg
	Cheese, Swiss	30 g (1 oz)	237 mg
	Sardines, canned	55 g (2 oz)	210 mg
	Cheese, Cheddar	30 g (1 oz)	209 mg
Good: 10-19% DV	Molasses, blackstrap	1 Tbsp	172 mg
	Cheese, mozzarella	30 g (1 oz)	151 mg
	Soybeans, cooked	90 g (~1/2 cup)	131 mg
	Collards, cooked	85 g (~1/2 cup)	119 mg
	Salmon, canned, with bones	55 g (2 oz)	117 mg
	Spinach, cooked*	85 g (~1/2 cup)	116 mg
	Turnip greens, cooked	85 g (~1/2 cup)	116 mg
	Black-eyed peas, cooked	90 g (~1/2 cup)	115 mg
	All Bran cereal	30 g (~1/2 cup)	100 mg

*In spinach, oxalate binds calcium and prevents absorption of all but about 5 percent of the plant's calcium.

Figure 11   Food Sources of Calcium.

Source: U.S. Department of Agriculture, Agriculture Research Service, 2003. USDA Nutrient Database for Standard Reference, Release 16. Nutrient Data Laboratory home page, http://www.nal.usda.gov/fnic/foodcomp.

intolerant (see Question 82), are amenorrheic, have higher than normal sweat rates, or are consuming a low-calorie diet. Athletes should bear in mind the following before taking a calcium supplement:

1. In order to maximize absorption, calcium should not be taken with other supplements. Iron and zinc compete with calcium, and if taken together, absorption rates will decrease.
2. Calcium supplements should be consumed with a small snack, as calcium is best absorbed when broken down by stomach acids first.
3. Calcium citrate is best absorbed by the stomach. Even though calcium carbonate has a higher amount of calcium, the calcium is not absorbed as well as calcium citrate. Calcium supplements produced from bone meal and/or oyster shells should be avoided as they may contain harmful levels of lead.
4. Less than 500 milligrams of calcium should be taken at one time; larger amounts can decrease absorption. If the athlete is required to take more than 500 milligrams per day, then it is recommended that the total be allotted over the entire day rather than at one time.

52. What is anemia, and how can it affect an athlete's performance?

Anemia is a condition that is characterized by a less than normal number of red blood cells in the blood or when the red blood cells do not have enough **hemoglobin** to carry oxygen. Iron is an essential trace mineral that is necessary in the formation of hemoglobin and myoglobin, which is an oxygen-binding pigment in the body (as shown in **Figure 12**), and for enzymes involved in energy production. When athletes are anemic

Anemia

A condition that occurs when less than the normal number of red blood cells are in the blood or when the red blood cells in the blood do not have enough hemoglobin.

Hemoglobin

A complex protein–iron compound in the blood that carries oxygen to the cells from the lungs and carbon dioxide away from the cells to the lungs.

Vitamins and Minerals

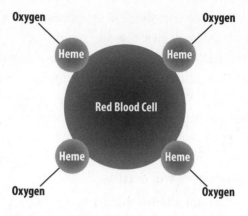

Figure 12   Red Blood Cell Binding with Oxygen.

(low in iron), they may feel tired and fatigue prematurely during exercise because of the reduced oxygen-carrying capacity of the red blood cells. Common causes and remedies of iron depletion are displayed in **Table 17**. Approximately 9% to 11% of female athletes are considered to be anemic. Although this is higher than the percentage of male athletes, male athletes, especially endurance athletes, are also susceptible to the condition.

Quick Fact

Because of the demands of their sports, endurance athletes are more susceptible to iron deficiency.

53. How long does it usually take to reverse anemia?

If an athlete has been diagnosed with anemia, it may take 3 to 6 months to reverse. All anemia cases should be monitored by a healthcare provider. The recommended treatment is typically 325 mg (with 65 mg of elemental iron) of ferrous sulfate, two to three times per day. Iron is a hard mineral to absorb, and thus, it should be taken between meals with a source of vitamin C

Table 17   Common Causes of Iron Depletion and Remedies to Improve Iron Status

Common Causes	Remedies
Inadequate energy intake.	Increase total calorie intake by consuming a well-balanced diet.
Avoidance of red meat, fish, and poultry that contain iron in the readily available **heme iron**.	Consume more sources of meat, fish, and poultry.
Iron intake solely from plant sources, **nonheme iron**, is harder to absorb than heme sources.	Include more heme sources of iron, but if the athlete follows a vegetarian diet, then increasing the amount of nonheme sources in the diet along with a source of vitamin C is necessary.
Increased iron losses in sweat, feces, urine, and menstrual blood.	These are unavoidable, but can be compensated for by increasing total calorie intake as well as increasing both nonheme and heme sources of iron.

Heme iron

A well-absorbed form of iron found in red meats, fish, and poultry.

Nonheme iron

A less well-absorbed form of iron found in fruits, vegetables, grains, and nuts.

H2 blockers

Anti-hypertensive medications that is used to control blood pressure.

Tea, coffee, calcium, antacids, H2 blockers (Pepcid, Zantac), and proton pump inhibitors (Prilosec, Nexium) may inhibit iron absorption; thus, avoiding these products when consuming foods high in iron or iron supplements will help maximize absorption.

(such as orange juice) to enhance its absorption. Tea, coffee, calcium, antacids, **H2 blockers** (Pepcid, Zantac), and proton pump inhibitors (Prilosec, Nexium) may inhibit iron absorption; thus, avoiding these products when consuming foods high in iron or iron supplements will help maximize absorption.

There are potential side effects when consuming larger than normal amounts of iron. The most prevalent side effect is constipation; if you experience this, consult with your healthcare provider. Athletes who have been diagnosed with anemia and are taking iron supplements need to get re-tested every 3 months until iron levels have returned to normal. Avoid taking iron supplements without a firm diagnosis of anemia (from your healthcare provider), as excess iron intake can be toxic to both the liver and heart. Athletes should not self-diagnose anemia.

Vitamins and Minerals

Fluids

Why should athletes consume water as part of their
nutrition plan?

Is thirst a good predictor of an athlete's fluid needs?

How much sweat can an athlete lose per hour
of exercise in a hot environment?

More . . .

What, when, and how much fluid an athlete consumes are critical to how an athlete performs. Hydration is often overlooked, but it plays a primary role in the equation for athletic success. Part Five identifies the signs and symptoms of dehydration and hyponatremia, provides the pros and cons of using sports beverages, and offers some excellent strategies for calculating individual fluid losses and fluid needs to help create a hydration plan.

54. Why should athletes consume water as part of their nutrition plan?

Water plays a critical role in an athlete's mental and physical performance. Water makes up approximately 60% of the body's weight and must be consumed regularly throughout the day to offset daily losses (urine, respiratory, and sweat). Athletes have a tendency to avoid consuming water throughout the day and generally focus on consumption during exercise. This inadequate consumption of fluids during the day potentially sets the athlete up for failure by creating a fluid deficit that may lead to poor physical and mental performance.

This failure to consume fluids is most likely the result of inaccessibility. This can be resolved effortlessly by advising the athlete to keep a water bottle handy for easy access and consumption. Water comes from fluids and foods, including tap or bottled water, juices, milk, sports drinks, fruits, and vegetables. **Table 18** shows the advantages of regular water consumption.

55. Is thirst a good predictor of an athlete's fluid needs?

Thirst is a poor predictor of an athlete's fluid needs. Athletes need to consume fluids on a regular basis

Table 18   Advantages of Water Consumption

1. Regulates body temperature (evaporative cooling)
2. Promotes waste product removal from the exercising muscle
3. Helps to prevent injuries
4. Lubricates joints
5. Maintains blood flow and oxygen to the exercising muscle
6. Aids in digestion
7. Optimizes muscle contraction
8. Decreases mental and physical fatigue

throughout the day and during exercise even if they do not feel thirsty. By the time the **thirst reflex** is felt, dehydration has already occurred, which can result in the athlete losing his or her competitive edge.

Thirst is caused by changes in blood sodium levels. When athletes sweat heavily, they lose more fluids than sodium from their bodies. The decreased **blood volume** results in an increase in **blood sodium concentration** (>130 mmol/L). This increased concentration promotes the human thirst reflex.

A useful tool for the athlete to determine his or her hydration status is to check on the color, frequency, and volume of his or her urine. When an athlete is well hydrated, urine color will be a pale, straw color (not clear) and frequent. Dark, concentrated urine that is low in volume and infrequent is generally an indication that the athlete needs to consume more fluids. Certain foods and vitamin supplements can change urine color, giving a false sense of hydration status.

Thirst reflex

A signal by the body to help regulate fluid balance.

Blood volume

Volume of blood circulating in a person's body. The blood consists of red blood cells and plasma.

Blood sodium concentration

Concentration of the amount of sodium in the blood. Normal levels are between 136 and 145 mmol/L.

56. How much sweat can an athlete lose per hour of exercise in a hot environment?

Athletes exercising in a hot environment can potentially lose as much as 2 to 3 pints of sweat per hour, which is approximately 2 to 3 pounds of body weight. Not only is the athlete losing water weight, but valuable electrolytes, particularly sodium, are lost as well. Fluid and electrolytes are replaced by consuming foods and fluids both during and after exercise.

The major constituents of sweat are water, sodium, chloride, potassium, iron, and calcium. For each liter of sweat lost during exercise, the athlete loses approximately 1,000 mg of sodium. Athletes engaged in endurance or ultraendurance events may lose as much as 1 to 2 liters (2 to 4 pints) of fluid per hour of exercise.

■ *Case Study*

Chris is a 37-year-old adventure racer with 9 years of experience. He has decided to compete in an adventure race in Florida where summer temperatures can reach 85°F or higher with relative humidity over 90%. Chris's primary concerns include preventing dehydration and ensuring adequate sodium replacement during the race. Chris recently completed a 1-hour laboratory **sweat test** to determine his sweat rate, electrolyte losses, and overall fluid needs. The results demonstrated that at a temperature of 80°F and 70% relative humidity, he lost approximately 1.1 liters (2 pints) of sweat and 950 mg of sodium during the hour. This sweat and sodium loss is similar to the established findings for endurance athletes (1 to 2 liters of sweat or 2 to 4 pints lost per hour and 1,000 mg of sodium lost per liter of sweat). This information was then used to design a drinking plan for Chris that will help prevent dehydration and provide enough sodium to eliminate the possibility of

Sweat test

A method to determine sweat rate, electrolyte losses, and overall fluid needs.

hyponatremia (see Question 65). Chris would be required to consume a commercial sports drink at a rate of 8 ounces every 15 to 20 minutes. The sports drink should contain at least 150 to 200 mg of sodium per 8 ounces, taste good, and help avoid stomach upset. At this rate of consumption per hour, Chris should be able to ingest close to the amount of fluid and sodium losses he typically experiences during exercise. Chris will be encouraged to gradually build his tolerance to the type and volume of fluid needed in order to maximize stomach absorption, helping to prevent dehydration and excess loss of sodium.

Quick Fact

1 pint = 2 cups

Quick Fact

1 liter = 2 pints

Quick Fact

1 teaspoon of table salt = 2,325 milligrams of sodium

57. How do I calculate my fluid needs?

Athletes can accurately estimate their fluid losses by weighing themselves before and after each workout. To ensure accuracy, athletes should weigh themselves in dry, lightweight clothing (or dry, nude weight) before and after exercise. After exercise, it is necessary for the athlete to dry all sweat completely from his or her body to guarantee an accurate post-exercise weight. For every pound (16 ounces/2 cups) lost, 24 ounces (3 cups) of fluid need to be consumed. The extra 8 ounces (1 cup) of fluid are needed to offset urinary and respiratory losses that continue after exercise. In rare instances, body weight

After exercise, it is necessary for the athlete to dry all sweat completely from his or her body to guarantee an accurate post-exercise weight.

may increase. If this occurs, the athlete may be consuming too much fluid (overhydrating) and will need to reduce fluid consumption. Failure to do so may lead to the dangerous condition of hyponatremia (see Question 65). Before the next workout, ensuring that weight has returned to pre-exercise levels guarantees that the athlete has achieved optimal hydration. If weight has not returned to a normal level, the athlete risks compromising future performance. Athletes who have not achieved their previous day's weight should be either barred from practicing or if allowed to practice, be carefully monitored for increased susceptibility to heat stress.

This method for determining fluid loss does not need to be conducted before and after every practice. After a drinking plan has been established, the athlete should be able to regulate his or her hydration status without having to weigh himself or herself continually.

Here is a formula for determining sweat loss:

Total sweat loss = pre-exercise weight *minus* post-exercise weight *minus* fluid consumed during exercise

■ *Case Study*

Tomas, a 21-year-old boxer, presents to the sports dietitian with feelings of dizziness and poor performance near the end of a 2-hour workout. He was asked to keep a 6-day log of his pre-exercise and post-exercise weights and the number of ounces of fluid consumed during each workout. **Table 19** presents the result of his 6-day weight and fluid log.

Quick Fact

A 2% drop in body weight, due to sweat loss, can decrease endurance by 6% to 7%.

Table 19 Results of Body Weight and Fluid Log

Day	Pre-Exercise Weight (Pounds)	Post-Exercise Weight (Pounds)	Fluids Consumed (Ounces)	Weight Loss (Pounds)	Water Loss (Ounces)
1	189.8	187.6	54	2.2	89.2
2	190.4	188.2	26	2.2	61.2
3	190.6	187.6	19	3	67
4	191.6	186.6	4	5	84
5	190.6	186.6	16	4	80
6	188.0	183.8	11	4.2	78.2
Averages	190.2	186.7	21.7	3.4	76.6

Fluids

190 pounds × 1% body weight loss = 1.9 pounds

190 pounds × 2% body weight loss = 3.8 pounds

190 pounds × 3% body weight loss = 5.7 pounds

Conclusions

Average sweat loss of approximately 2% body mass during workout

Average loss of 76.6 ounces of fluid per 2 hours of exercise

Average loss of 38.3 ounces of fluid per 1 hour of exercise

The goal is for Tomas to consume 30 to 40 ounces of fluids per hour (8 to 10 ounces every 15 to 20 minutes) of exercise to ensure optimal hydration and performance.

58. What is an example of a drinking plan?

An athlete must develop a drinking plan before, during, and after every practice or competition. Being prepared and drinking the right fluids, in the right amounts, at the right times, can mean the difference between a mediocre or successful performance. Individuals have different fluid requirements and tolerances; ranges are provided in **Table 20**.

Table 20   Typical Drinking Plan

Before practice/competition: Consume 8 to 16 ounces (1 to 2 cups) of fluid 15 to 30 minutes before exercise.
During practice/competition: Consume 5 to 12 ounces (0.5 to 1.5 cups) of fluid every 15 to 20 minutes.
After practice/competition: Consume 24 ounces (3 cups) of fluid for every pound lost.

59. Does the temperature of fluids consumed affect the rate of absorption from the stomach?

Contrary to popular belief, the temperature of fluids consumed before, during, or after exercise does not influence the rate at which they are absorbed from the stomach. Cold beverages are not absorbed any faster into the bloodstream than beverages drunk at room temperature. Cooler fluids have a tendency to be consumed

Quick Fact

Although cold beverages consumed during exercise have no impact on absorption, they may help cool the core temperature down by using metabolic heat to warm the fluid. This helps to reduce the amount of heat having to go to the skin's surface for evaporative cooling, reducing the rate of fluid loss and dehydration.

at higher rates, 40% to 80% more, than warmer beverages because of greater **palatability**. The temperature of the consumed fluid will depend on the personal preference of each athlete.

Stomach absorption is influenced by the volume of the fluid consumed and its caloric content. The greater the volume of fluid consumed, the faster is the rate of absorption. The optimal volume of fluid absorbed from the stomach is approximately 600 milliliters (2.5 cups) in the average athlete. Exceeding the 600-milliliter range has the potential to cause gastrointestinal issues and vomiting. Consuming less than 600 milliliters slows the rate of absorption and may negatively affect the athlete's hydration status. A higher caloric content (greater than 8% carbohydrate) can slow the rate of absorption, delaying fluid delivery into the circulation.

60. What should I look for in a sports drink?

Sports drinks are designed to provide three basic needs: hydration (water), energy (calories), and electrolytes (sodium, chloride, and potassium). An athlete should look for a drink that provides a 4% to 8% carbohydrate solution, meaning approximately 15 grams of carbohydrates (50 calories) per 8 ounces. A solution that is less or greater than the recommended 4% to 8% may reduce its effectiveness, causing gastrointestinal problems and delaying **gastric emptying**. **Figure 13** represents a modified sports drink label to assist the athlete in understanding what the essential ingredients are in a sports drink. The athlete should look for a drink that has 12 to 18 grams of carbohydrate, 0 grams of fat, and 0 to 4 grams of protein per serving. Fat and protein will delay stomach absorption and should be limited during exercise. For those athletes who have a hard time staying hydrated, a sports drink that contains

Palatability

Acceptable taste or flavor.

Fluids

An athlete should look for a drink that provides a 4% to 8% carbohydrate solution, meaning approximately 15 grams of carbohydrates (50 calories) per 8 ounces.

Gastric emptying

The rate at which foods and fluids exit the stomach.

117

Nutrition Facts:

Serving Size: 8 ounces (1 cup)

Amount Per Serving

Calories: 50–80

Total Fat: 0 g

Sodium: 100–200 mg

Potassium: 30–50 mg

Total Carbohydrate: 12–18 g

Protein: 0–4 g

Figure 13   Modified Sports Drink Label.

a small amount of protein (0 to 4 grams per 8 ounces) may help the athlete achieve a better hydration level. This type of formula should be tested during practice to determine individual tolerance and to avoid potential gastrointestinal problems.

Electrolytes are lost in sweat and must be replaced in order to optimize the athlete's hydration status. Sodium is the most abundant electrolyte lost in sweat. Sodium losses can exceed 1,000 milligrams per liter of sweat during vigorous activity. Sodium has numerous functions in athletic performance that include helping to retain fluid in the circulation (expanding blood volume), stimulating thirst (increasing frequency of fluid consumption), adding palatability (taste) to the beverage, and helping to reduce muscle cramping. The recommended amount of sodium per 8-ounce serving should range between 100 and 200 milligrams in order for it to be effective. Some athletes may exceed this requirement, as they may be heavy sweaters and therefore lose larger amounts of sodium in their sweat

Electrolytes

Potassium, chloride, and sodium are found in sweat. They are needed to maintain normal metabolism and function. For example, sodium is essential in maintaining fluid balance.

than the average athlete. Athletes who find themselves to be heavy sweaters should consider a laboratory sweat test to help determine how much sodium and sweat they are losing during 60 minutes of exercise at 70% VO_2 max (at 80°F and 50% relative humidity).

Some additional considerations when choosing a sports drink include taste (sweet, salty, sour, bitter), flavor intensity (weak or strong), appearance (appealing or unappealing), texture (thin or thick), and the fact that taste buds change during exercise. A variety of formulas and flavors of sports drinks exist on the market to satisfy each athlete's unique personal preference. Athletes should take the time to experiment with the various beverages on the market to help determine what works best for them.

Quick Fact

Remember to take your own sports drinks with you to races or competitions. Usually, the race will provide you with some type of sports drink, but it may not be one that you like or can tolerate. Before the event, check the website to determine what brand of fluid will be provided.

Not all sports drinks are created equal; therefore, read the label carefully and consult with a registered dietitian if you have any additional concerns or questions.

Quick Fact

Watch out for additives to sports drinks (minerals, vitamins, herbals) as well as the unsubstantiated claims about their potential benefits. Recent research has shown that the addition of vitamin C has no impact on performance, B vitamins actually decrease palatability of the beverage, and vitamin E increases inflammation.

61. Should sports drinks be diluted?

Sports drinks should not be diluted with water (or any other beverage). Sports drinks are specifically designed to replace lost energy, electrolytes, and fluids during and after exercise. Diluting sports drinks may reduce their effectiveness, delaying recovery and negatively impacting the next workout. Weaker solutions deliver less sugar to the intestine from the stomach, reducing the amount of energy reaching the circulation and working muscle. If a 6% solution is diluted in half to 3%, an athlete would be required to consume twice the volume of fluid to get the same energy value as found in the 6% solution. This has the potential to delay restoration and recovery of hydration status and glycogen stores because of stomach overload.

■ *Case Study*

Zoe, a female volleyball player, reports to the sports dietitian complaining of low energy during workouts. Zoe reports consuming 32 ounces of sports drink per workout and is confused about why she is experiencing premature fatigue. On further investigation, the dietitian finds that Zoe has been diluting the sports drink with water because she heard from teammates that sports drinks will cause weight gain. For every 8 ounces of sports drink, Zoe adds an additional 8 ounces of water. This dilution results in half the recommended amount of calories and carbohydrates being consumed, thus reducing the amount of energy available to her exercising muscles. For every 8 ounces of diluted sports drink consumed, Zoe is only getting 25 calories and 7.5 grams of carbohydrate versus the formulated amount, which contains 50 calories and 15 grams of carbohydrate per 8 ounces. This deficit is likely the cause of her early onset of fatigue. The sports dietitian recommends that Zoe stop diluting the sports drink, and within a few days, Zoe reports that her fatigue has subsided. She does not need to be concerned with weight gain, as the energy demands of the sport far exceeds the calories consumed from the sports drink.

62. Can energy drinks be used in place of sports drinks?

Many athletes have been led to believe that **energy drinks** have the same value as sports drinks in that they provide hydration, energy, and increased athletic performance. Energy drinks are *not* sports drinks. Energy drinks should *not* be used for hydrating before, during, or after exercise because of their potential side effects. Unlike a traditional sports drink that contains a 4% to 8% carbohydrate concentration, energy drinks exceed the upper end of the limit to values of 12% or higher. This greater concentration of carbohydrate in the stomach leads to larger amounts of fluid being pulled from the circulation with the potential to cause dehydration and potential gastrointestinal upsets leading to diarrhea and vomiting. Other side effects may include dehydration from increased urinary output, nausea, stomach cramps, rapid heart rate, increased blood pressure, nervousness, irritability, and decreased concentration, and may lead to increased susceptibility to heat stress. Athletes should also be careful with products that contain additional ingredients, such as minerals, vitamins, caffeine, and herbal additives. Ingesting large quantities of these beverages may lead to decreased athletic performance and cause serious negative health consequences.

Adam's comments:

During my first year in college, my physical fitness level was high. With the stress of collegiate life, by my junior year, I had gained over 30 pounds. My fitness level had dropped appreciably, and I felt I was heading down what seemed

Energy drinks

Drinks that advertise that they will improve physical and mental performance. Many add caffeine, vitamins, and herbal supplements that often act as stimulants.

Fluids

like a never-ending spiral. I needed some help and needed it fast. Not only is health important, but because I'm in the military, it is part of my job. I consulted with a sports dietitian and exercise physiologist to help me get back on track and get within military body fat and fitness standards. I was educated in the right way to lose weight, maintain health, and increase personal fitness. I found out that my personal way of losing weight was actually doing more harm than good. With my old program, I was not only not getting enough calories throughout the day, but I was exercising too much without getting adequate recovery.

I was baseline tested for my body fat (BodPod), cardiorespiratory fitness (VO_2 max test), and daily nutrition program. After this initial assessment, I was counseled on proper weight loss, and an exercise program was designed with my specific physiological parameters. After less than 12 weeks of doing the program, I dropped almost 10 pounds, and over 90% of the weight lost was fat mass. Not only did I drop fat and get leaner, but I also improved my cardiovascular fitness tremendously by reducing my mile and a half run time by 90 seconds. I am grateful for the opportunity to have worked with two professionals who showed me how sports nutrition and exercise science could help me improve the quality of my life.

Central nervous system

Body system that consists of the brain and spinal cord.

Alcohol is a central nervous system depressant and should not be consumed by anyone under the age of 21 years.

63. What are the effects of alcohol on athletic performance?

Alcohol is a **central nervous system** depressant and should not be consumed by anyone under the age of 21 years. A drink is considered to be 12 ounces of beer, 4 ounces of wine, or 1 ounce of spirits. Research has shown that potential health benefits are associated with moderate consumption of alcohol. Moderate consumption is no more than one drink per day for women and no more than two drinks per day for men. The health benefits, however, are not a reason for an individual to start consuming alcoholic beverages. For athletes, alcoholic beverages should not be consumed less than 12 hours before competition or practice, as the **diuretic** effects of alcohol can still be felt as long as 24 hours after consumption. **Table 21** identifies some of the more common causes and effects of alcohol consumption.

Diuretic

A drug or other substance that tends to promote the formation and excretion of urine.

Quick Fact

The negative effects of alcohol consumption may be felt as long as 48 hours after consumption.

Table 21 Cause and Effects of Alcohol Consumption on Athletic Performance

Cause	Effects
Diuretic	• Promotes fluid loss from the body by increasing urinary output leading to dehydration.
Central nervous system depressant	• Causes decreased performance because of the delayed reaction time, reduced mental focus, and poor coordination leading to increased injury potential.
Decreased muscle blood flow	• Reduces blood flow to exercising muscles, decreasing energy production and waste product removal. • Postpones muscle recovery after exercise, resulting in premature muscle fatigue, injury, and decreased performance • Reduces glycogen and protein synthesis.
Sedative	• Interrupts rapid eye movement (REM) sleep, causing increased daytime sleepiness, resulting in inadvertent napping. • Additionally, decreases focus and attention resulting in increased injury potential.

Fluids

64. What are the signs and symptoms of dehydration?

Dehydration occurs when there is an excess loss of water from the body, leading to a negative fluid balance. Water is found primarily in the circulation, between and inside body cells. The primary ways in which water is lost from the body include sweating, urination, respiration, and occasionally diarrhea and vomiting. When water loss exceeds water intake, dehydration occurs.

There are two different types of dehydration: voluntary and involuntary. **Voluntary dehydration** normally occurs when an athlete ignores the need to drink, has a poor thirst reflex, and/or refuses to carry a water bottle and consume fluids before and during exercise. Some athletes involved in sports with weight classifications, such as wrestlers, boxers, rowers, and jockeys, will intentionally withhold fluids to meet weight requirements of the sport. **Involuntary dehydration** occurs when the athlete does not have control over his or her fluid consumption or the rate at which the fluids can be lost and absorbed. This often happens when an athlete's sweat rate exceeds his or her ability to consume and absorb fluids from the stomach into the circulation. Some athletes are sometimes unable to access fluids on a consistent basis because of the demands of their sport. A soccer player is a good example of an athlete who may involuntarily dehydrate. Soccer players are required to be on the playing field for 45 minutes each half (90 minutes per game), which makes it difficult for the player to access the necessary amount of fluids needed to maintain his or her hydration. It has been demonstrated that soccer players, in hot environments, can lose as much as 2 to 3 liters (4 to 6 pints) of sweat per game determined by their pre-exercise

Dehydration

A condition resulting from a negative water balance (i.e., water loss exceeds water intake).

Voluntary dehydration

Normally occurs when an athlete ignores the need to drink, has a poor thirst reflex, and/or refuses to carry a water bottle and consume fluids before and during exercise.

Involuntary dehydration

When an athlete does not have control over his or her fluid consumption or the rate at which the fluids can be lost and absorbed.

weight and post-exercise weight. Athletes can see how involuntary dehydration can be detrimental to their physical and mental performance. For athletes in similar situations, the most opportune time to be able to consume fluids would be before the game and during half-time, as well as during injury and substitute time-outs.

Urine color and frequency are strategies that can easily be used by athletes to determine their hydration status. Urine should be pale, straw colored, and frequent, indicating optimum hydration levels. If urine is dark yellow and infrequent, this may indicate dehydration. Be aware that some vitamins can cause urine to be dark and odorous, giving a false sense of hydration status. An athlete's hydration goal should be to have a need to urinate before and after practice or competition. The lack of need indicates that the athlete is most likely in a state of dehydration and may feel some of the symptoms identified in **Table 22**.

When sweat is lost, vital electrolytes are lost as well. During and after exercise, electrolyte replacement can be accomplished by the consumption of a well-formulated sports drink.

Ways to prevent dehydration include the following:

1. Consuming fluids regularly throughout the day; begin early and drink often.
2. Avoid consuming large amounts of fluids at one time; avoid playing catch up.
3. Consume more salty foods or add more salt to foods.

Athletes need to identify the more common signs and symptoms of dehydration and should be aware that they may not experience all of these symptoms

Table 22   Signs and Symptoms of Dehydration

Decreased appetite
Difficulty concentrating
Dark, concentrated urine
Low urine volume
Nausea and vomiting
Restlessness
Swollen hands and feet
Lethargy
Confusion
Agitation
Headache
Seizures
Increased risk of injury
Decreased muscle strength and speed
Dry, cracked lips

simultaneously. Athletes should be aware that their fluid needs are based on their level of physical activity and surrounding environment. The hydration continuum chart (**Figure 14**) details various activity levels against fluid requirements.

Quick Fact

Be aware that certain drugs or supplements may contain ingredients that cause involuntary dehydration.

Fluids

Hydration Continuum

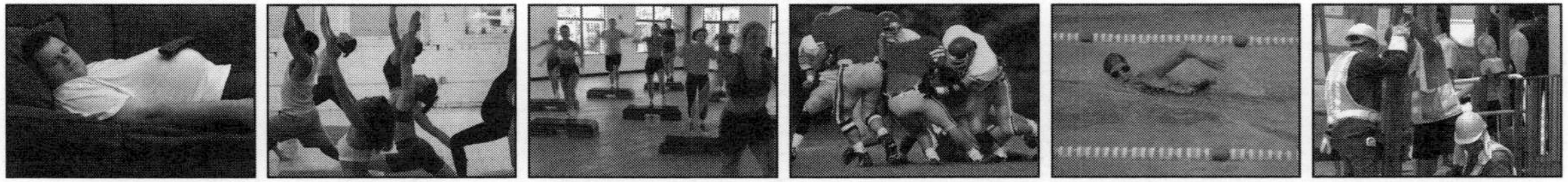

	Sedentary (24 h)	Low-intensity Short-duration (30 min)	Moderate-intensity Moderate-duration (60 min)	High-intensity Moderate-duration (60–120 min)	Moderate-intensity Long-duration (2–8+ h)	Low-intensity Long-duration (8+ h)
Typical Sweat Loss*	0 ml	0–0.5 L	0.5–1.5 L	1.0–3.0 L	1.0–16.0+ L	2.0–12.0+ L
Typical Sodium Loss**	1.5–3.0 g	0–0.5 g	0.5–1.5 g	1.0–3.0 g	1.0–16.0 g	2.0–12.0 g
Drink Schedule	2.0–4.0 L/d	0–0.5 L	0.5–1.5 L	1.0–3.0 L	1.0–15.0 L	2.0–12.0 L
Beverage Type	water coffee tea milk fruit juice soft drinks soup	nothing water fitness water sports drinks	nothing water fitness water sports drinks	sports drinks water	sports drinks water extra sodium	sports drinks water coffee tea milk fruit juice soft drinks soup

* = typical sweat rates for most people under most conditions; some may sweat more
** = assumes a loss of 1.0 g sodium per liter of sweat (43 mmol Na+/L)

Figure 14   Hydration Continuum.

Source: Courtesy of Dr. Bob Murray, Sports Science Insights, LLC *Photos:* Spauln/Shutterstock, Inc.; Photodisc; Ryan McVay/Photodisc/Getty Images; Photolink/Photodisc/Getty Images; Photodisc; Christinee/Dreamstime.com.

> ### Quick Fact
>
> Intravenous fluid replacement is generally warranted for athletes who have lost approximately 7% or more of their total body weight as sweat. This usually occurs when an athlete has difficulty keeping fluids in the body because of vomiting and/or diarrhea.

65. What is hyponatremia, and why should athletes be concerned about it?

Hyponatremia

A lower than normal concentration of sodium in the blood, caused by inadequate excretion of water or by excessive water in the circulating bloodstream.

Hyponatremia (overhydration) is a potentially life-threatening condition that occurs when an athlete's blood sodium concentration drops to less than 130 mmol/L. To help avoid this potentially life-threatening condition, the athlete must maintain an adequate electrolyte balance during exercise. Athletes become susceptible to hyponatremia when they replace sweat losses with water only or consume excessive amounts of water before exercise. Hyponatremia is more commonly encountered in endurance athletes who are exercising or competing for several hours at a time or athletes who are sweating more than normal because of warm environmental conditions.

Hyponatremia is often mistaken for dehydration because many of the symptoms are similar. The most distinctive symptoms are the color, volume, and frequency of urine. Athletes who are hyponatremic will have light-colored urine, a high urine output, and frequent urination, whereas those who are dehydrated will have dark-colored urine, a low urine output, and infrequent urination.

Hyponatremia is treated by correctly identifying that it is occurring. The seriousness of the case must be professionally diagnosed. Medical monitoring is required to determine whether an athlete is able to hold foods and fluids down and/or whether the athlete is conscious or unconscious. The treatment will depend on the level of severity and can include consuming fluids or foods that contain sodium or by intravenous fluid treatment and not by increasing water consumption.

An athlete needs to be aware of the signs and symptoms of hyponatremia (**Table 23**) and recognize that he or she may not experience all of these symptoms simultaneously.

Table 23   Signs and Symptoms of Hyponatremia

Decreased appetite
Difficulty concentrating
Light-colored urine
High urine volume
Nausea and vomiting
Restlessness
Swollen hands and feet
Lethargy
Confusion
Agitation
Headache
Seizures
Increased risk of injury
Decreased muscle strength and speed

Weight Management

How do I recognize a fad diet?

What constitutes body composition?

What role do body mass index, waist circumference, and waist-to-hip ratio play in my performance?

More . . .

Part Six discusses weight issues that include proper weight loss and weight gain, eating disorders, and body composition measurements and methods. This section provides guidance regarding the importance of sensible weight management for athletes, coaches, teammates, and parents.

66. How do I recognize a fad diet?

Fad diets

Weight-loss programs or supplements that promise to deliver quick weight loss with minimal effort.

The long-term use of fad diets has led to dangerous conditions that include dehydration, proteolysis (muscle protein loss), hypotension, and possible liver and kidney failure.

Fad diets are weight-loss programs or supplements that promise to deliver quick weight loss with minimal effort. Fad diets are appealing to some athletes, as time is always a factor, but the negative implications on performance are not worth the risk. Fad diets are not supported with scientific research; therefore, the claims made regarding the products and/or ways of eating are not proven to be healthful or effective over the long term. The long-term use of fad diets has led to dangerous conditions that include dehydration, proteolysis (muscle protein loss), hypotension, and possible liver and kidney failure. Most fad diets are unmanageable, and the short-term weight loss is usually gained back once the athlete no longer or is unable to follow the diet. Weight loss is usually water and glycogen loss, and it is counterproductive to athletic performance by causing dehydration and early onset of fatigue. The best way to distinguish a fad diet from a healthful program is to recognize these important characteristics. Fad diets usually do the following:

1. Recommend eliminating or limiting certain foods or food groups.
2. Claim weight loss of greater than 1 to 2 pounds per week.
3. Sound too good to be true.

4. Promise that you will not have to modify your diet at all, meaning that you can eat unhealthy foods and still lose weight.

5. Have dramatic pictures, exaggerated statements, and claims.

6. Necessitate that you must buy the product in bulk, purchase meals or shakes, or attend seminars for the plan to be successful.

7. Have studies that are not reviewed by other researchers.

There is no quick and easy way to lose weight; weight loss is a gradual process that requires dietary and exercise modifications, consistency, and patience in order to achieve long-term success. Although some fad diets are popular and may "work" for a short time, the repercussions far outweigh the temporary benefits.

67. What constitutes body composition?

Body composition is comprised of **fat mass** and **fat-free mass**. Fat mass is the composition of fat in the body that includes fat stored in the cells and **essential body fat**. Fat mass is categorized as either essential or non-essential. Essential body fat is the fat associated with the internal organs, central nervous system, bone marrow, mammary glands (females), and pelvic region (females), whereas non-essential body fat is found in **adipose tissue**. Essential body fat is vital for proper functioning of the body and should not drop below 5% in males and 12% in females. Fat-free mass is the weight of all body components except fat and is primarily made of the skeletal muscles (minerals, protein, and water) and organ weight. Approximately 70% of fat free mass is comprised of water compared with only 10% in fat mass.

Weight Management

Fat mass

The portion of body composition that is fat. Fat mass includes both fat stored in the fat cells and essential body fat.

Fat-free mass

The weight of all body substances except fat. Fat-free mass is primarily made of organ weight and the skeletal muscles, including minerals, protein, and water.

Essential body fat

Fats found within the body that are essential to the normal structure and function of the body.

Non-essential body fat

Fat found in adipose tissue. Non-essential body fat is also called "storage fat."

Adipose tissue

Made of adipocytes, which store excess dietary fat not used by the body.

Quick Fact

Fat-free mass and lean body mass are often used interchangeably. The difference between the two is that lean body mass includes essential fat and fat-free mass does not.

Percent body fat

The amount of fat mass found on the body expressed as a percentage of total body weight.

Percent body fat is the percentage of total body weight that is fat mass. The body fat percentage is often used by athletes, coaches, trainers, sports dietitians, exercise physiologists, and doctors to assess an athlete's optimal health and performance.

Body composition varies among athletes and can be affected by the specific sport, gender, age, genetics, activity level, dietary intake, disease, and injury. For young athletes who begin a sport before puberty, it is important to understand that maturation may have positive or negative implications for their particular sport. During pubertal growth, changes occur in both adipose and muscle tissue, not always welcomed by athletes in all sports. Athletes who compete in aesthetic sports, such as gymnastics, often have a hard time adjusting to the increase in body fat during maturation because their sport emphasizes low body weight, a petite frame, and low body fat.

Some athletes (boxers, wrestlers, rowers, divers, ballerinas, figure skaters, and jockeys) desire to compete at low weight categories in order to gain a competitive advantage. Body composition, when used appropriately, can be a useful tool to determine whether competition is realistic at a lower weight category. Methods for assessing body composition can be found in Question 69. Body composition assessment can play an important role in successful athletic performance, but it should not be overly stressed. If body composition, namely body fat percentage, is overemphasized, it could lead to disordered eating or eating-disordered behaviors.

68. What role do body mass index, waist circumference, and waist-to-hip ratio play in my performance?

Body mass index (BMI), **waist circumference**, and **waist-to-hip ratio** are often used to measure fitness, body size, and body composition. Individually, these numbers do not always provide the most accurate picture; however, when used together as part of a comprehensive evaluation, these assessments can provide a dependable guideline to help athletes determine a healthy weight that will positively contribute to their sports performance.

BMI is calculated from the athlete's height and weight measurements; BMI equals the weight in kilograms per height in meters squared. The calculated number is then compared with the BMI ranges that have been set by the National Heart, Lung, and Blood Institute, shown in **Table 24**.

BMI has some limitations, as it is not gender or race specific and does not correlate well for all athletes. BMI often classifies athletes with higher amounts of

Table 24   BMI Ranges

Classification	BMI
Underweight	<18.5
Normal weight	18.5–24.5
Overweight	25–29.9
Obesity (Class I)	30–34.9
Obesity (Class II)	35–39.9
Extreme Obesity (Class III)	>40

Weight Management

Body mass index (BMI)

An indicator of nutritional status that is derived from height and weight measurements. Body mass index has also been used to provide a rough estimate of body composition even though the index does not account for the weight contributions from fat and muscle.

Waist circumference

A measure of abdominal girth taken at the narrowest part of the waist as viewed from the front.

Waist-to-hip ratio

A comparison of waist girth to hip girth that gives an indication of fat deposition patterns in the body.

muscle mass as overweight even though they are healthy and physically fit. These factors must be taken into consideration, and BMI data must be used in conjunction with other assessment methods to evaluate body composition and fitness accurately.

> ## Quick Fact
>
> 1 kilogram = 2.2 pounds, 1 inch = 2.54 centimeters, 100 centimeters = 1 meter

What is the BMI of an athlete who is 69 inches tall and weighs 155 pounds?

BMI = weight in kilograms/height in meters squared

Weight: 155 pounds/2.2 kilograms = 70.5 kilograms

Height: 69 inches × 2.54 centimeters = 175.2 centimeters

175.2 centimeres/100 = 1.752 meters

BMI = 70.5 kilograms/(1.752 meters)^2 = 20.1 (normal weight)

The waist-to-hip ratio compares waist (abdominal circumference) to hip girth to determine whether body fat is deposited in the upper or lower part of the body.

Waist circumference is a simple way to measure body fat distribution. Body fat distribution is a strong predictor of chronic disease (cardiovascular, diabetes, hypertension) and mortality. Waist circumference is measured by taping (measuring) the smallest part of the waist. An unhealthy waist circumference is defined as greater than 40 inches in males and greater than 35 inches in females. Waist circumference is often used in conjunction with BMI to predict associated health risks that are seen in **Table 25**.

The waist-to-hip ratio compares waist (abdominal circumference) to hip girth to determine whether body

Table 25   Classification of Overweight and Obesity by BMI and Waist Circumference, and Associated Disease Risk*

Weight Classification	BMI (kg/m²)	Obesity Class	Men ≤ 102 cm (≤40 in) Women ≤ 88 cm (≤35 in)	Men > 102 cm (>40 in) Women > 88 cm (>35 in)
Under-weight	<18.5	—	—	—
Normal†	18.5–24.9	—	—	—
Over-weight	25.0–29.9	—	Increased	High
Obesity	30.0–34.9	I	High	Very high
	35.0–39.9	II	Very high	Very high
Extreme obesity	≥40	III	Extremely high	Extremely high

*Disease risk for type 2 diabetes, hypertension, and CVD.

†Increased waist circumference can also be a marker for increased risk, even in persons of normal weight.

Source: National Heart, Lung, and Blood Institute, National Institutes of Health, U.S. Department of Health and Human Services. Clinical Guidelines on the Identification, Evaluation, and Treatment of Overweight and Obesity in Adults, Evidence Report, 1998. NIH Publication No. 98-4083.

fat is deposited in the upper or lower part of the body. The waist-to-hip ratio is the waist (smallest part of the waist) divided by the hip (taken around the hips and over the buttocks where the greatest girth is found). A waist-to-hip ratio of more than 0.95 inches for males and more than 0.80 inches for females increases the risk of diseases, including cardiovascular, particular cancers, diabetes, and hypertension. **Figure 15** depicts the android (apple) versus gynoid (pear) fat distribution patterns found in men and women.

Athletes can effectively apply these simple measuring techniques to help monitor their weight fluctuations and distributions.

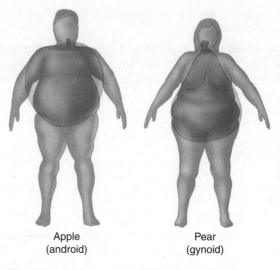

Apple
(android)

Pear
(gynoid)

Figure 15   Apple versus Pear Shape Patterns in Men and Women.

69. What is a body composition assessment? What are the various methods available to compute body composition? What is their accuracy?

Body composition assessment measures the percentage of fat mass and lean body mass. It can be an important tool in helping an athlete to achieve his or her ideal weight to optimize performance. A lack of lean body mass impedes strength and endurance and increases susceptibility to injury. To improve lean body and reduce fat mass, it is important for an athlete to engage in a scientifically designed sports-specific nutrition and exercise program. Athletes who carry too much body fat for their sport may experience decreased performance through compromised speed, agility, premature fatigue, and injury. To help design an effective nutrition and exercise program, athletes should consider consulting with a registered dietitian and exercise physiologist for professional guidance.

Body composition differs between men and women. Average body fat levels for men are between 15% and 18%, and 22% and 25% for women. Athletes are often lower than the average ranges but should not fall below 5% for men or 12% for women. Falling below these ranges can lead to potential health consequences that include diminished bone density, a reduction in testosterone levels in males, and decreased estrogen and progesterone levels in females. Many athletes, depending on their sport, have levels that are significantly lower or higher than the average and should be aware that letting body fat levels exceed the ranges may negatively impact health and athletic performance. Body composition directly correlates with sports performance. Several studies have shown that higher body fat adversely affects maximal aerobic capacity and performance during endurance events.

There are several body composition assessment methods, and the availability and accuracy of each method used to compute body composition will vary. Because of the sophistication of some of these devices, their availability and cost can be prohibitive. **Table 26** provides an overview of the methods of body composition assessment.

70. What part of the season is the appropriate time for an athlete to lose or gain weight?

An athlete should not intentionally try to gain or lose weight during the **in-season**. Weight changes should be addressed in the **off-season**. Changing body composition during the in-season could have detrimental effects on performance. Unintentional fluctuations in body weight (up or down) during the in-season may be an indication that the athlete is consuming too few or too

In-season
Part of the training schedule that consists of a high amount of activity and competition.

Off-season
Part of the training schedule that consists of less than the normal amount of activity.

Table 26 Common Methods of Body Composition Assessment

Assessment Method	Description	Accuracy	Accessibility
Hydrostatic weighing (underwater weighing)	This is the gold standard of body composition determination that involves weighing a person while he or she is totally immersed in water.	High	Low
Plethysmography (BodPod)	This technique measures the volume of air displaced by an object or body. In body composition assessment, air displacement plethysmography is used to determine the volume of the body so that the body density can be determined.	High	Low
Skinfold calipers	This instrument is used to measure the thickness of skin folds in millimeters.	Medium	Medium-High
Bioelectrical impedance analysis	This body composition assessment technique measures the resistance to flow of an insensible electric current through the body; the percentage of body fat is then calculated from these impedance measurements.	Low-Medium	Low
Dual-energy X-ray absorptiometry	This method of body composition is an assessment that involves scanning the body using radiography technology to distinguish between fat and lean body tissue.	High	Low
Circumference method	This method uses height, weight, and various body locations that are then compared with a standard table. Women and men are measured at the following sites: women: neck, waist, hip; men: neck, waist.	Medium	High

many calories for his or her activity level. Weight loss incurred during the in-season often results in the loss of both muscle mass and fat mass, which may lead to poor performance and increased potential for injury.

■ *Case Study*

Andy, a college wrestler, presents to the sports dietitian at the beginning of the season with a goal of cutting weight in order to wrestle in a lower weight class. Andy's body fat is at 8% (males should not be less than 5% body fat for performance and health reasons), and his weight is still 7 pounds above the weight limit. The sports dietitian is concerned that Andy's weight loss may impede his performance because the season has already begun and Andy does not have much fat mass to lose. Andy is 200 pounds at the beginning of the season; the 7-pound weight reduction would put Andy below the 5% body fat minimum. This means that Andy would have to lose an additional 1 pound of lean body mass to stay above the 5% range. Knowing that Andy must lose lean muscle mass in order to make the lower weight class, the sports dietitian does not recommend that Andy wrestle at the lower weight class. Andy should also be discouraged from trying to make the lower weight by dehydrating himself (excess exercise, saunas, rubber suits). This common dehydration practice to losing weight can have serious health and performance consequences for the athlete. Competing at the lower weight class is most likely going to affect his wrestling performance and recovery adversely. This goal weight would have been better achieved during the off-season when more time could be dedicated to healthy weight reduction by changing his training and nutrition regimen.

71. What are the recommendations for helping athletes to lose weight?

Athletes should lose weight during the off-season, at a rate of no more than 2 pounds per week, in order to help maintain lean body mass. In-season weight loss is discouraged, as it may negatively impact the athlete's performance. For athletes to lose 1 pound of fat mass per week, they would need to reduce calorie intake by

500 calories per day. In order to lose 2 pounds per week, a reduction of 1,000 calories per day would be required. If the goal is to lose more than 2 pounds per week, athletes should consult with a sports dietitian and/or healthcare provider for guidance.

The recommended limit of 2 pounds per week for weight loss may not be suitable for all athletes. Body size, percentage of body fat, and the sport requirements are all factors that must be taken into consideration before a weight-loss program is initiated. **Table 27** shows a comparison of an endurance athlete and a strength athlete who desire to lose 10 pounds.

Quick Fact

Too much weight loss or food restriction has been shown to impair immune function.

■ *Case Study*

Bryan, a 36 year old, 5'9", and 197 pound, professional firefighter reported to his physician complaining of chest discomfort after participating in the fire department's annual physical fitness assessment. Bryan was unable to complete the run portion of the test resulting in a fitness requirement failure. Additionally, Bryan measured 3 percent over the body fat limit necessitating that he lose weight in order to be able to continue his job safely and effectively. Bryan also complained that he was having a difficult time falling and staying asleep at night. After a thorough check-up, it was determined that Bryan had a moderate muscle strain of his pectoral muscle that needed rest and ice treatment only. Bryan's physician noticed that his blood pressure and cholesterol were mildly elevated potentially related to his poor dietary habits, weight gain, and infrequent exercising. Bryan was referred to a registered dietitian and an exercise

Table 27 Comparison of an Endurance Athlete's and a Strength Athlete's Weight-Loss Goals

Athlete	Marathon Runner	Football Player
Height	72 inches	72 inches
Weight	180 pounds	275 pounds
Body fat percentage	12%	20%
Goal	−10 pounds	−10 pounds
Time	4 weeks	4 weeks
Daily caloric consumption	3,000 calories/day	5,000 calories/day
Recommendations	1. Requires at least 5 weeks to lose weight because weight loss is not recommended at more than 2 pounds per week in order to maintain lean muscle mass. 2. A calorie deficit of 1,000 calories per day is needed to see this weight reduction of 2 pounds per week. 3. For this marathon runner, a 1,000 calorie per day reduction (33% of daily calories) would significantly impact his or her training performance. A better option would be to reduce caloric intake by 500 calories (16% of daily calories) per day over 10 weeks for safer weight loss to occur with less impact on performance. 4. Performance, recovery, and hunger cues must be monitored in order to ensure safe weight loss.	1. Requires at least 5 weeks to lose weight because weight loss is not recommended at more than 2 pounds per week in order to maintain lean muscle mass. 2. A calorie deficit of 1,000 calories per day is needed to see this weight reduction of 2 pounds per week. 3. For this football player, a 1,000 calorie (20% of daily calories) reduction per day would not significantly impact his training or performance. 4. Performance, recovery, and hunger cues must be monitored in order to ensure safe weight loss.

physiologist for help in developing a weight loss and exercise conditioning program.

The dietitian evaluated Bryan's 3-day food log and it revealed that he consumed the majority of his calories at breakfast. This was usual practice by the department's firemen; the reasoning behind this practice was to "stock up" on as many calories as possible in order to hold the firefighters over for the rest of the day, especially when they were busy on an emergency. The majority of Bryan's calories were coming from fat and protein in the form of eggs, ham, sausage, and hash browns. The dietitian noticed that Bryan rarely consumed fruits and vegetables and typically ate two large meals per day. The registered dietitian helped Bryan design a program that complimented his work schedule. The goals included balanced meals and consuming smaller and more frequent meals and snacks throughout the day.

Bryan also made an appointment with the exercise physiologist. During his visit he realized that his current exercise program was insufficient, in both duration and frequency, to meet the minimum requirements of the department's cardiorespiratory component of the fitness test. The exercise physiologist designed a progressive aerobic conditioning program for Bryan, requiring him to run 3 to 4 times per week for 30 minutes and then gradually progress to 60 minutes per session. In addition, a strength training program was designed to help Bryan develop both general and task specific strength that would help improve his firefighting skills and enhance weight loss.

After 12 weeks, Bryan returned to his physician 14 pounds lighter with a 4% decrease in body fat. Additionally, his blood pressure and total cholesterol had dropped significantly. Bryan was sleeping better at night and acknowledged that he had more energy throughout the day and less mental stress. Bryan repeated the department's fitness test and passed all components successfully.

Bryan's success motivated the department to establish a heart-healthy menu that offered an array of fruits and vegetables, wholegrain carbohydrates, and lean protein choices. The department also purchased some weights and a couple of treadmills to help promote a convenient means of remaining physically fit for their demanding job.

72. What are some effective strategies for gaining lean body mass?

Athletes who wish to gain weight for their sport should do so in the off-season when there is sufficient time without negatively impacting performance. Appropriate weight gain requires a sports-specific strength-training program in addition to a well-designed dietary plan that focuses on positive energy balance. To be in a positive energy balance, the athlete must consume more calories than he or she needs. The athlete's weight gain goals should be aimed at increasing muscle mass in order to keep a high strength-to-weight ratio. A high strength-to-weight ratio implies that the athlete has a high percentage of lean body mass for his or her absolute weight. If athletes fail to follow a well-designed strength and nutrition program, they may not be able to keep the strength-to-weight ratio high enough, leading to an excess gain in fat weight and possibly decreasing performance.

Appropriate weight gain requires a sports-specific strength-training program in addition to a well-designed dietary plan that focuses on positive energy balance.

Quick Fact

1 pound of fat mass = 3,500 calories. 1 pound of lean body mass = 2,800 calories.

A healthy weight gain is considered to be approximately 0.5 to 1.0 pound per week and can be accomplished by increasing daily caloric intake by 300 to 500 calories per day, decreasing energy expenditure, or combining the two.

Weight Management

In contrast to popular belief, gains in muscle mass occur gradually and require a moderate as opposed to a large intake in calories. Weight gains should be monitored by frequent body composition analysis in order to ensure that muscle rather than fat is being gained. Athletes should monitor their own progress by gauging how they are feeling and performing during workouts. If weight gain is rapid or if an athlete is not eating the appropriate number of calories, then the athlete may feel tired and sluggish, and performance may decrease. Rapid weight gain (over 0.5 to 1.0 pound per week) is not advisable, as the weight gained will most likely be fat. The additional calories should come from carbohydrates, *not* proteins, as some athletes believe. Carbohydrates are needed for energy and help prevent **gluconeogenesis** (the use of proteins to make glucose). A lack of carbohydrates in the diet can result in proteins being broken down for energy rather than being used for muscle growth (synthesis). This protein utilization will prevent gains in muscle mass. An increase in overall protein intake, in conjunction with an overall increase in calories, may be required for those athletes who are participating in intense strength training. An athlete's protein needs may increase to approximately 1.4 to 2.0 grams per kilogram of body weight under these circumstances. The increased protein can easily be achieved through a higher calorie intake as opposed to using protein supplements. Consuming excess protein can be harmful to the kidneys, and protein that is not used can be stored as fat.

Gluconeogenesis

The formation of glycogen from fatty acids and proteins rather than from carbohydrates.

Quick Fact

Weight gain has a strong genetic component; some athletes have a harder time gaining weight than others, even when following a proper strength and nutrition program.

Athletes are often concerned about the sensation of fullness when engaging in a weight-gain program. In order to prevent feeling overly full, athletes should consume foods and fluids frequently throughout the day (rather than eating three big meals), choose energy-dense foods, eat before drinking at mealtimes, and replace some whole grains with refined white products for quicker digestion.

The following tips are helpful for those athletes who are trying to gain weight:

1. Increase calorie intake by 300 to 500 calories per day; additional calories should come from carbohydrate (50% to 60%), protein (15% to 20%), and fat (20% to 30%) sources.

2. During intense strength training phases, protein needs may rise to 1.4 to 2.0 grams per kilogram. These needs can usually be met through dietary increases rather than supplements.

3. Try to consume three meals plus two to four snacks per day (include pre-exercise and post-exercise snacks) rather than three large meals. This is easily accomplished by consuming foods and fluids every 2 to 3 hours.

4. Do not skip snacks before bedtime. Snacks should include both carbohydrates and proteins. Because the body recovers during sleep, it is important to ensure that it has enough fuel to build and repair properly.

5. Choose energy-dense foods that provide more calories but will not be overfilling. Examples include smoothies, trail mix, dried fruits, nut butters, fruit juices, homemade milk drinks, and Carnation Instant Breakfast drinks.

6. Eat before you drink; do not fill up on beverages at meals, as this will cause premature fullness. Carbonated beverages may cause gas and bloating, leading to premature fullness.

7. Replace some whole-grain foods with refined white products to increase digestion and the desire to eat more frequently (every 2 to 3 hours).

8. Increased calorie needs for weight gain do not give the athlete free reign to consume large amounts of junk food (cookies, pastries, chips, etc.). A well-balanced diet will ensure gradual muscle mass gains rather than excess fat gains.

9. Engage in a regular strength training program at least three times per week to ensure gains in muscle mass.

73. What are the dangers to the athlete if body fat percentage drops too low?

Low body fat

Body fat levels below 5% for males and 12% for females.

Low body fat is a condition in which body fat levels drop below safe limits, creating the potential for adverse health outcomes. Body fat levels that are too low can be detrimental to both an athlete's health and performance (**Table 28**). The female athlete should not allow body fat levels to drop below 12%, and the male athlete should not allow drops below 5%. Although these are the current recommendations, there is variability among sports and individuals. These numbers are only general guidelines and not absolutes.

Some sports necessitate that athletes maintain a very low percentage of body fat for performance and aesthetic reasons. Sports that require low body fat levels include, but are not limited to, gymnastics, figure skating, wrestling, swimming, boxing, cross-country running, track and field, diving, rowing, volleyball, and ballet. Athletes in

Table 28   Negative Effects Associated with Low Body Fat Levels

Negative Effects
Diminished bone density (possible osteoporosis)
Increased incidence of stress fractures
Irregular menstrual cycle (females only)
Reduced circulating testosterone levels (males only)
Depressed immune function
Decreased absorption of fat soluble vitamins (A, D, E, and K)
Loss of insulation (leading to potential shivering/hypothermia)
Decreased protection of internal organs and muscles
Poor physical and mental performance

these sports are more susceptible to disordered eating and eating disorders, as they try to keep their body fat levels low. Athletes should be carefully monitored by coaches, parents, teammates, physicians, and sports dietitians in order to help prevent eating disorders.

74. What is an eating disorder, and what athletes might be at risk for an eating disorder?

Disordered eating is often the precursor to eating disorders. Disordered eating is observed when athletes alter their eating patterns, in an unsafe way, in an attempt to lose weight or maintain weight at a lower than normal weight. Disordered eating patterns often develop into eating disorders that are classified as anorexia nervosa, bulimia nervosa, or eating disorder–not otherwise specified. Although the highest prevalence of eating disorders is seen in adult females 18 to 30 years old, eating disorders affect millions of female and male athletes every day. It is estimated that among male and female athletes the incidence of eating disorders is 10% to 20%.

Disordered eating

Observed when athletes alter their eating patterns, in an unsafe way, in an attempt to lose weight or maintain weight at a lower than normal weight.

The intense focus on weight often leads to a negative body image and unhealthy eating behaviors that have grave health and performance consequences.

The intense focus on weight often leads to a negative body image and unhealthy eating behaviors that have grave health and performance consequences.

Certain sports or the culture around certain sports places some athletes at higher risk for disordered eating and eating-disordered behaviors. The American College of Sports Medicine developed a list of sports that are most likely to put athletes at risk, but these are not the only sports in which an athlete may develop an eating disorder.

1. Sports in which the athlete is judged based on aesthetics, including gymnastics, diving, figure skating, and ballet.
2. Sports in which the uniforms are required to be tight, revealing, or minimal, including swimming, volleyball, water polo, track, diving, gymnastics, ballet, figure skating, and cross-country.
3. Sports in which body fat is seen as a barrier to performance and a lean body type is stressed, including endurance sports such as triathlons, running, and cycling.
4. Sports in which weigh-ins and weight classifications are required, including rowing, wrestling, horse racing, boxing, weight lifting, and martial arts.

Other risk factors for eating disorders include individual versus team sports; influences of coaches, parents, siblings, and/or teammates; low self-esteem; family dysfunction; families with eating disorders; chronic dieting; a history of physical or sexual abuse; family or cultural pressures to be thin; and other traumatic experiences. Eating disorders are much more responsive to early intervention and treatment, as untreated eating disorders are insidious and potentially life-threatening. Seeking specialized care by a team consisting of registered

dietitians, medical doctors, and psychologists is important to help the athlete get on the right track to a healthy
lifestyle and improved performance.

75. What are the most common eating disorders?

Eating disorders are medical illnesses and are classified
into three groups: anorexia nervosa, bulimia nervosa,
and eating disorder not otherwise specified. The major
classifications are defined by the American Psychiatric
Association.

Anorexia nervosa is characterized by starvation and
extreme weight loss that is manifested by an extreme
fear of becoming obese, a distorted body image, and
avoidance of food. Anorexia nervosa can be life threatening and requires medical and psychiatric treatments.

Behaviors and symptoms of anorexia nervosa include
the following:

1. Refusal to maintain weight at or above minimally
   normal weight for height, body type, age, and
   activity level
2. Intense fear of weight gain or being "fat"
3. Feeling "fat" or overweight despite dramatic weight
   loss
4. Distorted body image
5. Loss of menstrual cycle
6. Extreme concern with body weight and shape

Bulimia nervosa is characterized by repeated and
uncontrolled bingeing in which a large number of calories are consumed in a short period of time, followed by
purging methods such as forced vomiting or use of laxatives or diuretics.

Weight Management

Anorexia nervosa

A clinical condition
manifested by
extreme fear of
becoming obese, a
distorted body image,
and avoidance of food.
Anorexia nervosa can
be life threatening
and requires medical
and psychiatric
treatments.

Bulimia nervosa

A clinical condition
characterized by
repeated and uncon-
trolled bingeing in
which a large number
of calories are con-
sumed in a short
period of time,
followed by purging
methods such as
forced vomiting or
use of laxatives or
diuretics.

Behaviors and symptoms of bulimia nervosa include the following:

1. Repeated episodes of bingeing and purging
2. Feeling out of control during a binge and eating beyond the point of comfortable fullness
3. Purging after a binge (vomiting, use of laxatives, diet pills and/or diuretics, excessive exercise, fasting)
4. Frequent dieting
5. Extreme concern with body weight and shape

Eating disorder not otherwise specified is an eating disorder that does not meet all of the criteria needed for it to be diagnosed as either bulimia nervosa or anorexia nervosa but that meets the criteria to be labeled as a true eating disorder. **Binge eating disorder** also falls under this category. It is characterized by recurrent episodes of binge eating, a lack of self-control during binge eating, and marked distress after a binge.

Behaviors and symptoms of eating disorder not otherwise specified include the following:

1. All the behaviors/symptoms of anorexia nervosa, except the athlete has a regular menstrual cycle
2. All the behaviors/symptoms of anorexia nervosa, but weight is in the normal range
3. All the behaviors/symptoms of bulimia nervosa, but binges are infrequent
4. Regular use of inappropriate compensatory behavior after eating small amounts of food

Several other disorders do not meet the criteria for a clinically defined eating disorder but are nevertheless still critical to recognize in order to prevent a more

Binge eating disorder

Falls under the category of eating disorder not otherwise specified. It is characterized by recurrent episodes of binge eating, a lack of self-control during binge eating, and marked distress after a binge.

serious problem: anorexia athletica, night eating syndrome, and muscle dysmorphia.

Anorexia athletica is seen in individuals who practice inappropriate eating behaviors and weight-control methods to prevent weight gain and/or fat increases. The characteristics of anorexia athletica include the following:

1. Decreased energy intake
2. Decreased weight in the absence of medical illness or affective disorder explaining the weight reduction
3. Maintenance of high physical performance
4. Desire to lose weight not based on appearance
5. Desired for weight loss based on performance or perceived performance improvements
6. Intense fear of weight gain
7. Weight cycling based on training levels
8. Dietary restraint
9. Bingeing and purging
10. Gastrointestinal complaints
11. Menstrual dysfunction
12. Compulsive exercise despite illness or injury
13. View self-worth by athletic ability to performance

Night eating syndrome is a disordered eating pattern that is characterized by 50% or more of total caloric intake eaten after 7 p.m., sleep disturbances, morning anorexia, and frequent eating during the night that lasts for over 3 months. Night eating syndrome is usually associated with overweight or obese individuals.

Muscle dysmorphia is a syndrome characterized by highly muscular individuals (usually men) having a

Weight Management

Anorexia athletica

A subclinical condition in which individuals practice inappropriate eating behaviors and weight-control methods to prevent weight gain and/or fat increases. Anorexia athletica does not meet the criteria for a clinically defined eating disorder, but the behaviors exhibited are on a continuum that could lead to the more severe clinically recognized eating disorders.

Night eating syndrome

A disordered eating pattern that is characterized by 50% or more of total caloric intake eaten after 7 p.m., sleep disturbances, morning anorexia, and frequent eating during the night that lasts for over 3 months. Night eating syndrome is usually associated with overweight or obese individuals.

Muscle dysmorphia

A type of disordered body image in which individuals have an intense and excessive preoccupation and/or dissatisfaction with body size and muscularity. Muscle dysmorphia is most prevalent in male bodybuilders and weight lifters.

pathological belief that they are small in nature. Athletes with this syndrome often demonstrate many of the same eating and exercise patterns as those who are anorexic or bulimic. The preoccupation with body shape and size frequently leads to avoidance of social situations and oftentimes the abuse of supplements and drugs to achieve body image goals.

Behaviors surrounding eating disorders are often secretive; thus, many go undetected. It is therefore important to be knowledgeable of the characteristics and behaviors of eating disorders in order to help prevent them from occurring. Prevention is the best defense.

76. How do eating disorders affect athletic performance?

Early stages of eating disorders falsely provide hope for athletes who suffer from this illness. In the early stages, athletes may see an increase in performance; however, this is short lived, and eventually performance will drastically decrease. Physical, mental, and behavioral changes occur, and the timeline for these changes differs for individual athletes. Some athletes are able to maintain their eating disorder behaviors longer than others without seeing significant adverse side effects; this, however, leads to more severe complications later. Complications associated with eating disorders include the following:

Some athletes are able to maintain their eating disorder behaviors longer than others without seeing significant adverse side effects; this, however, leads to more severe complications later.

1. Impaired physical and mental performance
2. Decreased concentration and chronic fatigue
3. Vitamin and mineral losses
4. Brittle nails and hair
5. Dry and yellow skin

6. Irregular menstrual cycle

7. Hormone imbalances

8. Inability to tolerate cold; presence of **lanugo**

9. Increased obsession with food, weight, and exercise

10. Decreased metabolic rate

11. Dental erosion

12. Decrease in lean body mass

13. Stress fractures/injuries

14. Low bone density

15. Dehydration, lightheadedness, dizziness, fatigue

16. Swollen salivary glands (neck)

17. Throat and/or stomach rupture

18. Sadness/depression

19. Glycogen depletion

20. Anxiety

21. Increased heart rate and damage to the heart muscle

22. Sleep disturbances

23. Gastrointestinal complications

The medical complications that arise as a side effect of eating disorders can be extremely severe. The athlete must get professional help from a registered dietitian, medical professional, and psychologist to help break the cycle, understand his or her hunger cues (see Question 2), and develop normal eating patterns.

77. What is the female athlete triad?

The **female athlete triad** is a group of three interrelated conditions—disordered eating, menstrual irregularities, and osteopenia/osteoporosis. It is typically diagnosed in young female athletes (**Figure 16**). Disordered eating often encompasses a negative self-body image and a conscious restriction of food. The lack of energy intake from

Lanugo

Fine, white hair that grows usually on the arms and chest of those who are severely underweight. The hair serves as a mechanism to keep the body warm where there is not enough body fat available to do so.

Female athlete triad

A group of three interrelated conditions, typically diagnosed in young female athletes—disordered eating, menstrual irregularities, and osteopenia/osteoporosis.

Weight Management

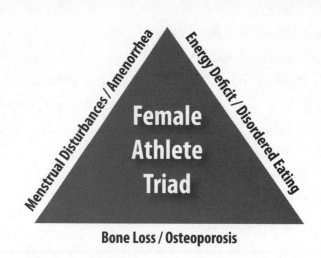

Figure 16 Female Athlete Triad.

disordered eating increases the likelihood of an irregular menstrual cycle and stress fractures that create serious health risks and medical concerns. All athletes are at risk if they are pressured to meet unrealistic weight and body fat goals set forth by coaches, teammates, parents, or the athlete himself or herself. The athletes who are most affected include those who are involved in aesthetic sports, sports with weight classifications, sports that require form fitting or minimal uniforms, and/or sports that stress low body fat percentages.

Thermoregulation

The control of heat production and heat loss for maintaining normal body temperature.

Disordered eating leads to an alteration in available energy; thus, if an athlete consumes less food (energy) than the amount required, energy levels will be inadequate to maintain physiological processes such as growth, reproduction, and **thermoregulation**. Altered physiological functioning can lead to impaired health and poor performance.

Eumenorrhea

A term used to describe normal menstruation consisting of at least 10 menstrual cycles per year.

Menstrual dysfunction is a result of low energy (calorie) intake. Normal menstruation, **eumenorrhea**, is when a female has at least 10 menstrual cycles per year. Cycles that differ from this norm are considered to be irregular: oligomenorrhea and amenorrhea. **Oligomenorrhea** is defined as four to six cycles per year. **Amenorrhea** is the absence of a menstrual cycle for more than three months or, in young female athletes, the delay in the age of menarche, which is 15 years old. These menstrual disturbances should be monitored closely, as hormonal changes can disrupt bone density.

Bone loss or osteoporosis is a result of low energy availability and menstrual irregularities. Loss of bone often results in **stress fractures** and can lead to early-onset osteoporosis.

The female athlete triad is seen in approximately 25% to 30% of the female athlete population. The symptoms include poor mental and physical performance, a loss of muscle mass, fatigue, anemia, electrolyte imbalances, recurrent injuries, and/or stress fractures. These health consequences often become chronic; therefore, prevention and early detection by athletes, parents, coaches, teammates, and medical professionals are crucial.

Oligomenorrhea

A condition in which the female menstrual period is irregular, with cycles occurring only four to six times per year.

Amenorrhea

The absence or abnormal cessation of menstruation; defined as less than four cycles per year.

Stress fractures

An overuse injury in which the fatigued muscle can no longer bear the stress and transfers it to the bone.

Weight Management

Quick Fact

Recent research has shown that the female athlete triad may actually be a tetrad: disordered eating, menstrual disturbances, loss of bone, and abnormal vascular function.

Extreme Environments

What are the effects of acute high-altitude exposure on performance?

What is the live-high/train-low concept?

What are the considerations for athletes training or competing in cold-weather ambient and/ or water environments?

More . . .

Environmental conditions can change abruptly for an athlete, negatively impacting his or her nutrition, hydration, and performance plan if not adequately educated and prepared. Part Seven raises the athlete's awareness regarding extreme environmental conditions with knowledge and strategies to help prepare and overcome environmental adversity.

78. What are the effects of acute high-altitude exposure on performance?

Many of today's athletes are required to compete in diverse environments, with high altitude being no exception. Sports such as cycling, trail running, and many alpine events are often conducted at altitudes of 8,000 feet or higher. Exercising at higher altitudes can place considerable demands on an athlete's pulmonary and cardiovascular systems. Athletes who fail to prepare adequately for high-altitude competition will be at a significant physical and mental disadvantage compared with athletes who spend the time and effort adapting.

Hypobaric

An environment, such as at high altitude, that involves low atmospheric pressure.

Atmospheric pressure

Force per unit area exerted against a surface by the weight of air above that surface. One atmosphere equals 14.7 pounds per square inch.

When an athlete is acutely exposed to a **hypobaric** environment, the body reacts by setting into motion a series of physiological responses to compensate for the diminished supply of oxygen at the tissue level (hypoxia). The pressure in the surrounding atmosphere decreases when an athlete enters a high-altitude environment. This reduction in **atmospheric pressure** results in less oxygen reaching the athlete's working muscles, which in turn causes a significant decline in aerobic capacity (VO_2 max). To compensate for the reduced oxygen availability at the tissue, the respiratory center of the brain is stimulated. This stimulation initiates an increase in rate and depth of respiration in an attempt to maintain sufficient oxygen to the lungs and circulation. Paradoxically, the increased respiratory rate at altitude will have little to no effect on pulmonary gas exchange and, therefore, no additional increases in oxygen delivery to the tissue. Without adequate atmospheric pressure to drive the oxygen into the blood and tissue, over breathing becomes ineffective.

In addition to increased lung ventilation, the athlete will also experience a rapid rise in both exercising and resting heart rate. This increase is a protective response required to push more blood and oxygen through the heart and blood vessels to compensate for the decreased atmospheric pressure and lower oxygen delivery to the tissue. The increase in **cardiac output** (amount of blood pumped by the heart each minute) and heart rate do very little to provide the tissues with additional oxygen because of the atmospheric pressure remaining compromised.

Cardiac output

The volume of blood being pumped by the heart in 1 minute: cardiac output = stroke volume × heart rate.

Athletes who are training to compete at high altitudes need a scientifically designed training plan to help them adapt to the detrimental effects of hypoxia. Adequate adaptation generally takes 2 to 3 weeks and requires the athlete to be exposed to high altitude every day during the training period. This regular exposure will help prevent many of the side effects— such as acute headaches, nausea, and dehydration— that are associated with exercise in a high-altitude environment. Regular exposure at a high altitude will eventually permit the athlete to expand his or her blood volume and increase the number of circulating red blood cells. These adaptations will provide the tissue with a greater supply of oxygen, thus permitting the athlete to compete at a higher level.

Athletes who are training to compete at high altitudes need a scientifically designed training plan to help them adapt to the detrimental effects of hypoxia.

79. What is the live-high/train-low concept?

Athletes having to compete at higher elevations are confronted with two important performance considerations: trying to compete within 24 hours of arriving at altitude or taking the time to gradually adapt. Competing within the first 24 hours helps to prevent symptoms of acute altitude sickness such as headache, nausea, and difficulty breathing; however, this is not always feasible, as it requires a significant amount of coordination and planning on the athlete's part. The alternative is to spend time living at the altitude (12 to 14 days) to allow the body to acclimate physiologically to the hypoxic conditions. This exposure facilitates the build up of red blood cells and helps to reduce the adverse effects of high-altitude competition (see Question 78).

Long-term exposure to higher elevations enables athletes to increase their VO_2 max values by as much as 5%; this is directly proportional to their red blood cell mass. This increase in aerobic capacity, however, does not necessarily translate into better performance. The lack of performance may be due to decreased training intensity at altitude, resulting from the athlete's reduced endurance capacity and cardiorespiratory function. In other words, physiologically, athletes may not be able to sustain a high enough training intensity at a high altitude to gain or even maintain their fitness. Ironically, the benefits of both high-altitude training and living can be negated by the decreased adaptation resulting from the reduced training intensity.

Recent studies have demonstrated the importance of the live-high and train-low concept. The premise allows athletes to gain the physiological benefits of high-altitude exposure in addition to maintaining the necessary training intensity at lower elevations. One study divided competitive runners into three groups: group 1 (high–low) lived at 8,200 feet and trained at 4,200 feet. Group 2 (high–high) lived and trained at 8,200 feet, and group 3 (low–low) lived and trained at 490 feet. The results of the study demonstrated that the high–low and high–high group had the same improvements in VO_2 max values; however, it was only the high–low group that showed an improvement in running performance. This study reinforces the need for athletes to be able to train with sufficient intensity to enhance performance.

As a result of the effectiveness of the live–high/ train–low concept, athletes sought an alternative to the high–low requirement. As a result, a few companies developed hypobaric tents or chambers as a way of circumventing the conventional method of exposure and adaptation. The concept behind the hypobaric tent is to gradually reduce the oxygen concentration of the breathable air and simultaneously increasing its nitrogen content, thus creating a hypobaric environment. The athlete then sleeps or rests in the tent for a required period of time, gaining the physiological benefits while eliminating the need for high-altitude exposure. To date, there have not been enough carefully controlled experiments demonstrating the effectiveness of hypobaric devices as a method for improving physiological capacity and performance.

In conclusion, there appears to be a definite benefit to living high and training low when it comes to performance enhancement; however, the time, cost, and discomfort associated with this method may not be feasible for all athletes.

Extreme Environments

80. What are the considerations for athletes training or competing in cold-weather ambient and/or water environments?

When athletes compete or train in cold-weather environments, greater demands are placed on their body's carbohydrate stores. The increased carbohydrate utilization results from the body burning additional energy to protect its **core temperature**, 98.6°F. A shivering athlete will expend approximately 60% of his or her body's total carbohydrate stores in order to help maintain the core temperature. This extra energy consumption can rapidly drain the cell's glycogen stores, leading to compromised performance that will likely result in premature mental and muscular fatigue. **Figure 17** represents the typical flow of energy expenditure during cold weather exercise.

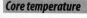

Core temperature

Temperature in the body's core, 98.6°F.

81. What impact can the heat have on my performance?

Athletes are frequently required to exercise or compete in high environmental temperatures. The 1996 Atlanta Olympics took place during the summer months, where average daily temperatures were in the high 80s and relative humidity was over 90%. Many athletes who competed in these games were coming from countries that had temperate climates. These extreme conditions can place tremendous physiological demands on the athlete.

The body produces heat during digestion, energy storage, respiration, and muscle contraction and is required to maintain its core temperature at 98.6°F. The body's temperature is carefully controlled through the process of thermoregulation, which is a mechanism that the body uses to control heat production and heat loss in order to maintain a normal body temperature.

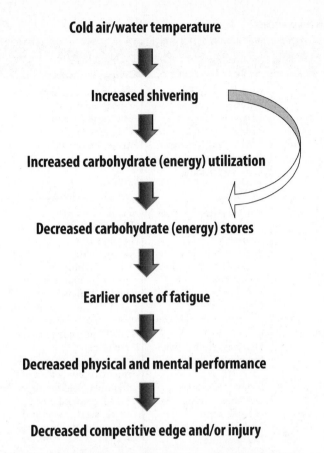

Cold air/water temperature

Increased shivering

Increased carbohydrate (energy) utilization

Decreased carbohydrate (energy) stores

Earlier onset of fatigue

Decreased physical and mental performance

Decreased competitive edge and/or injury

Figure 17   Flow of Energy Expenditure During Cold-Weather Exercise.

An athlete exercising in a hot, humid environment can overload his or her body with excess heat causing mild to severe reactions (**Table 29**).

> ## Quick Fact
> Thirty percent of the muscle's energy is used directly for muscular contraction. The remaining 70% is lost in the form of heat.

Athletes exercising in hot and/or humid environments will experience an increase in core temperature because of heat being released from within the muscles

Extreme Environments

Table 29   Heat-Related Disorders

Heat-Related Disorder	Degree of Severity	Signs and Symptoms	Corrective Actions
Heat cramps	Mild	Muscle cramping Excessive sweating Irritability Mild dizziness, weakness Prickly heat (tiny red bumps on the skin also cause a prickling sensation)	Rest in a cool, shaded area Stretch muscle Moderate activity Consume fluids Keep skin dry and clean
Heat exhaustion	Moderate	Profuse sweating Cold, clammy skin Faintness Weakness, fatigue Headache, nausea, loss of appetite Rapid pulse Hypotension	Cease activity Rest in a cool, shaded area Lie down Consume fluids Use cool compresses on forehead and neck and under armpits
Heat stroke	Severe	Lack of sweat Dry, hot, flushed skin Deep, rapid breathing Irregular, weak pulse Headache, nausea Decreased muscle coordination Mental confusion Disorientation Loss of consciousness Convulsions	Call for immediate medical attention Rest in a cool, shaded area Initiate cooling of the body (fanning, cold towels, or ice packs around the neck, under arms, and groin) Immerse or douse in cold water Consume fluids (if conscious)

Combustion

A process that produces heat.

(energy **combustion**) and absorption from the external environment. As core temperature rises, heat is conducted to the circulating blood, which is then shunted to the surface of the skin through vasodilation of the skin surface blood vessels. This increased skin blood flow stimulates sweat glands to release sweat to the skin's surface. As sweat gathers on the surface of the skin, it evaporates to the surrounding environment, removing heat and cooling the body. Athletes who exercise in humid conditions are more susceptible to thermal strain because of less sweat evaporating from the body. When the moisture content in the air is equal to or greater than the athlete's skin moisture, a barrier is created, leading to a cessation of sweat evaporation. This loss of evaporation can lead to an increase in core temperature and a greater susceptibility to heat-related disorders.

Quick Fact

For every gram of sweat that evaporates from the skin's surface, 0.6 calories of heat are removed with it.

Athletes who sweat excessively during exercise are highly susceptible to acute dehydration. Athletes who fail to replace lost fluids regularly can experience a rapid onset of fatigue resulting from a diminished blood volume and, therefore, blood flow to the exercising muscle. As water is removed from the bloodstream for evaporative cooling and is not replaced through drinking, the blood volume will decrease, resulting in blood becoming more viscous (thicker). The increased blood thickness reduces the amount of blood able to go to and from the heart and exercising muscle, increasing an athlete's RPE for the same workload. The heart's response to this reduction in blood flow to the muscle is to increase heart rate (number of beats per minute) in order to compensate for the blood's higher viscosity. This is often referred to as cardiac drift. Cardiac drift can be minimized by the frequent consumption of fluids (see Question 54).

There are many factors for athletes to consider when exercising in hot and/or humid environments:

1. Acclimation: It is important for athletes to expose themselves progressively to a hot environment. It takes

approximately 10 to 14 days for a non-acclimated athlete to adjust to a hotter climate. During this time, athletes must gradually increase their exercise intensity and duration to maximize adaptation reducing the potential for thermal strain.

2. Consume plenty of fluids: Drink water and sports drinks at regular intervals throughout the day and especially during exercise.

3. Take frequent breaks as needed: Do not be ashamed to slow down or rest in the shade. When the air is still, sweat tends to drip rather than evaporate from the body, reducing heat loss. To promote evaporative cooling, athletes can fan themselves using an electric or manual fan.

4. Wear proper clothing: Wear loose, lightweight, sweat absorbent clothing (see Question 41).

5. Maintain fitness: Muscles that are well conditioned generate less body heat. Excess body weight taxes the body more by producing larger amounts of heat and sweat. Athletes with higher cardiovascular fitness acclimate to hot environments faster.

6. Eat right: Consume small, frequent meals and snacks throughout the day, and ensure that the foods being consumed have enough salt in them to replace the salt lost through sweat. Using extra salt at mealtimes can be beneficial for those athletes who are heavy sweaters.

7. Age: Be aware that younger and older athletes are more susceptible to heat stress.

8. Unique threats: The risk of heat stress increases with the intake of alcohol, caffeine, and certain medications (high blood pressure, allergy medicines). Medical conditions (diabetes) and recent illnesses (flu) also increase susceptibility to heat stress.

■ *Case Study*

Nina, a 19-year-old collegiate field hockey player, has returned to school for pre-season practices. It is late August, and the temperature has been in the mid-80s with a relative humidity of 85%. After the third day of pre-season practice, Nina presents to the athletic trainer with cold, clammy skin, a rapid heart rate, dizziness, and disorientation. The athletic trainer suspects a case of possible heat exhaustion.

On further investigation, the athletic trainer realizes that Nina had spent the 3 months of summer vacation in the Northwest, where daily temperatures were in the upper 70s with moderate humidity. Because she has only been back to school for a few days, where the temperatures are hot and humid (more than she is used to), her body is not yet acclimated to the hotter environment. Although Nina had been training over the summer and is in good cardiovascular shape, it still takes approximately 10 to 14 days to acclimate fully to the new environment. Unfortunately, Nina was unable to acclimate gradually because pre-season two-a-day practices started the day after she returned to school. Nina told the trainer that breaks have been limited during workouts, and she has been unable to consume sufficient fluid during practices. After practices, she makes a concerted effort to consume fluids but has noticed her appetite has been low; also, she has not been able to consume much food. The athletic trainer sends Nina to meet with the sports dietitian who recommends the following:

1. Consume fluids on a regular basis throughout the day and during exercise by carrying a water bottle. Sports drinks are highly recommended because of the high fluid, energy, and electrolyte losses during two-a-day practices in a hot, humid environment.

Extreme Environments

2. Consume smaller, more frequent meals and snacks throughout the day. It is important for the athlete to remain well fueled. If appetite remains low, it is critical for the athlete to seek medical attention to rule out the possibility of a more serious medical condition.

3. When breaks are provided, try to rest in a shaded area, if possible. Breaks are also the perfect time to consume fluids and carbohydrates.

4. Between and/or after practices, resting in a cool environment is imperative. It is recommended to stand in front of a fan, if provided in a field setting, or in an air-conditioned space, if indoors.

5. Nina will not have time to acclimate fully during the week-long pre-season practices because she was unable to return to school more than one day before training commenced. She must understand that if she feels any of the symptoms again, she must cease activity immediately and report back to the trainer. The goal is to prevent another episode of heat exhaustion and possibly a more severe case of heat stroke.

PART EIGHT

Nutritional and Exercise Considerations for Special Populations

What is lactose intolerance?

What is the overtraining syndrome?

How do I know whether my decreasing performance over the season is related to overtraining or poor nutritional habits?

More . . .

Lactose intolerance

The body's inability to digest significant amounts of lactose (sugar found in milk and other dairy products) because of low or absent levels of the enzyme lactase.

Lactose

A sugar found in milk that is composed of glucose and galactose.

Lactase

A digestive enzyme that breaks lactose into the simple sugars glucose and galactose.

Galactose

A simple sugar found in milk.

Food allergy

Occurs when the immune system attacks a food protein and produces an adverse reaction such as itching, hives, rash, swelling, labored breathing, and/or loss of consciousness.

Food intolerance

Irritation of the digestive system when a food is unable to be broken down.

Immune system

A system within an organism that protects against disease.

Part 8 provides information for athletes who have special requirements based on age, gender, and dietary restrictions caused by personal, medical, and/or travel circumstances. The fundamentals of sports nutrition and exercise remain primarily the same, with a few minor modifications for these athletes. Awareness and implementation of these modifications will help an athlete with special requirements avoid unnecessary performance obstacles.

82. What is lactose intolerance?

Lactose intolerance is the body's inability to digest significant amounts of **lactose** (sugar found in milk and other dairy products) because of low or absent levels of the enzyme **lactase**. Lactase is produced in the stomach and is necessary to break down lactose into two simple forms of sugar, glucose and **galactose**, which can then be absorbed into the bloodstream.

Lactose intolerance is not a **food allergy**; it is a **food intolerance** in the digestive system. Lactose intolerance is not a reaction triggered by the **immune system**. Symptoms of undigested lactose include nausea, cramps, bloating, gas, and diarrhea. Symptoms can be mild to severe and usually begin within 30 minutes to 2 hours after ingestion of foods containing lactose. The severity of symptoms can be influenced by several factors that may include the amount of lactose a person can tolerate, speed of digestion, age, and ethnicity.

Between 30 and 50 million Americans are considered to be lactose intolerant. The most susceptible populations include African Americans, Native Americans, and Asian Americans.

Lactose intolerance is easily treated through the diet. Individuals should understand what dairy products they can and cannot tolerate and in what amounts. Knowing this information can help in establishing a dietary plan that includes both dairy and non-dairy products. Particular individuals may be able to tolerate small amounts of dairy products without any side effects, whereas others may react to even the smallest amount. Those who are able to tolerate small amounts can usually control their symptoms through diet alone. Those who are unable to tolerate small amounts of lactose can purchase over-the-counter lactase enzymes (such as lactaid pills) or lactose-reduced or lactose-free food products.

Calcium intake is a nutrition concern for those unable to tolerate dairy products. Calcium is essential in building and repairing bone tissue and is required for muscle contraction and the maintenance of blood calcium levels; therefore, athletes with lactose intolerance who are unable to consume dairy products must eat other foods that contain calcium. Some excellent sources of calcium include dark green leafy vegetables, salmon, sardines, yogurt, and calcium-fortified soy milk. Calcium supplements are recommended in some cases, although individuals should check with a healthcare provider before beginning any supplement.

83. What is the overtraining syndrome?

Overtraining syndrome is generally described by coaches and athletes alike as a condition that results in a steady decrease in physical and mental performance over time. Athletes have expressed subjective feelings of constant tiredness, persistent muscle and joint soreness, an inability to focus, and/or feeling burned-out or stale. Overtraining is very difficult to diagnose, as there is no definitive way to test for it. Many of the symptoms of overtraining can be similar to certain medical and

Overtraining syndrome

A condition that results in a steady decrease in physical and mental performance over time. Symptoms include constant tiredness, persistent muscle and joint soreness, inability to focus, and/or feeling burned-out or stale.

psychological conditions. There is an array of potential symptoms associated with the overtraining syndrome; however, no two athletes will experience identical signs.

One of the chief causes of overtraining is a lack of sufficient recovery or rest between intense or frequent training sessions. Athletes who find themselves engaged in repetitive high-intensity training workouts or who train every day without adequate recovery are likely candidates for the overtraining syndrome. High-intensity training is necessary for an athlete to develop maximal strength, speed, and power, a concept often referred to as overreaching or supercompensation. After several days of intense training, the athlete should follow up with a few days of reduced training intensity and volume to allow the body to adapt and recover. Failure of the athlete to incorporate sufficient recovery between training days can result in maladaptation, resulting in burnout and possible injury. To help avoid the overtraining syndrome, coaches often employ strength and conditioning specialists to assist athletes in the development of **periodized** training programs that incorporate regular fluctuations in training intensity and volume. These periodized training programs integrate scientific principles of exercise that include intensity, frequency, duration, and specificity. The correct application of these principles has been very effective in helping athletes avoid overtraining.

Periodized

A phased program that allows the body to adapt and recover in order to achieve optimal gains.

After an athlete is considered to have overtraining syndrome, very little can be done other than total rest to overcome the problem. There have been cases in which some athletes have never fully recovered from the effects of overtraining. Athletes and coaches need to be educated on the potential signs and symptoms of overtraining and request professional medical intervention if they suspect that it is occurring. The sooner the coach and athlete seek help the less chance there is that the athlete will succumb to the overtraining condition. As a preventative measure, coaches and athletes should request the help of an exercise physiologist and sports dietitian to ensure that the athlete's training and diet programs are providing adequate recovery and performance nutrition.

Some of the potential signs and symptoms of overtraining include the following:

1. Decreased performance and higher rating of perceived exertion at the same workload
2. A loss of appetite
3. Persistent muscle and joint soreness
4. Unexplained weight loss and inability to gain weight
5. Increased susceptibility to infection and illness
6. Poor mental focus
7. Constant feelings of fatigue
8. An inability to fall and stay asleep
9. Possible increases in resting heart rate
10. Feeling of depression, irritability, and anger

A multitude of symptoms are associated with overtraining syndrome, and if athletes experience a few of these symptoms for any period of time, they should consult with their healthcare provider to rule out possible medical complications. The multidisciplinary approach involving the physician, exercise physiologist, sports dietitian, sports psychologist, coach, and the athlete is a more successful approach to treating and preventing overtraining syndrome than either approach alone.

84. How do I know whether my decreasing performance over the season is related to overtraining or poor nutritional habits?

Sport-specific nutrition is usually one of the most neglected aspects of an athlete's training program. What an athlete eats immediately before, during, and after practice or competition can be critical to how the athlete performs not only that day, but also in the weeks and months to come. It is vital that an athlete properly fuel his or her body. A car cannot be expected to work without the right type of gas; similarly, one cannot expect his or her body to run efficiently without the right fuel (foods/fluids) either. Athletes must be careful to realize that not all foods are created equal; there is not just one "super food" that will allow them to perform optimally.

■ *Case Study*

Jade is a 16-year-old water polo player who has been playing the game for 4 years. She loves water polo and wants to compete at the collegiate level, but she is regularly plagued by a recurring injury around mid-season. Most mornings Jade finds herself physically and mentally exhausted, getting up only a few minutes before the bus arrives. Because she wakes up late, she rarely eats breakfast. A few hours after arriving at school, Jade begins to feel hungry and has a difficult time concentrating in class. By lunch time, Jade's hunger is intense. To satisfy her hunger and low energy level, Jade often chooses to eat a grilled-cheese sandwich, fries, and an energy drink. After school, Jade heads to practice for a 2-hour workout without eating or drinking anything immediately before, during, or after practice. Jade's next meal is at home about 1.5 hours after practice ends. After dinner with her family, Jade does her homework. When finished, she watches television and then heads to her room to instant message some of her friends before going to bed. Before Jade realizes it, it is 11 p.m., and she is physically and mentally exhausted. Jade falls asleep quickly, and before she knows it, the alarm clock is ringing. She wakes and comments, "It feels like I just fell asleep." Jade rolls over and hits the snooze button to get some additional sleep, but realizes that she never feels fully rested from her night's sleep.

She has fallen into a cycle that is causing her to feel worse as the season progresses. On top of feeling worse, Jade realizes that over the weeks and months of the water polo season, she feels more worn down and exhausted. Jade even finds herself falling asleep in class and wanting to skip practice to get extra rest. Jade has noticed that it is becoming more difficult to maintain her energy and focus during practice and in school. At the beginning of the season, 2-hour practices went by quickly; now, every minute seems to drag.

Jade's mother noticed that Jade continues to be mentally and physically exhausted and that her injuries continue to plague her. She also noticed that she regularly skips breakfast and rarely brings food to eat on the bus. She took Jade to the physician who suggested that some of Jade's problems may be directly related to her poor nutritional habits. The physician suggested that Jade and her mother make an appointment to meet with a sports dietitian.

The sports dietitian helped Jade develop a nutrition plan that would keep her mentally and physically focused for both school and water polo. Simultaneously, the plan would speed up the recovery of her nagging injuries. Together, they reviewed Jade's current eating and drinking schedule to evaluate its effectiveness. This is what they discovered:

1. Jade is frequently skipping breakfast to get extra sleep.
2. Jade is overly hungry at lunchtime and often chooses inappropriate meals that do not enhance her performance in the classroom or at afternoon water polo practice.
3. Jade does not consume any foods or fluids immediately before, during, or after practice.
4. Jade waits too long after practice to eat her next meal.
5. Jade is not getting enough sleep.

The recommendations for Jade are as follows:

1. Jade must consume meals and snacks that are high in carbohydrates regularly throughout the day in order to have the energy she needs to stay alert in class and play her best.
2. Jade should regularly consume energy (through meals and snacks) so that she will not be overly hungry at any one time and be able to choose foods that are performance enhancing rather than performance decreasing.
3. With the help of a sports dietitian, Jade developed a customized eating and drinking plan that she can follow before, during, and after practices/games. Timing of meals and snacks is imperative for optimizing Jade's performance and recovery.

Although Jade appears to be experiencing symptoms of the overtraining syndrome, in actuality, she is suffering from poor dietary habits. After implementing the recommended sports nutrition strategies, Jade began to feel more energetic during the school day and practice. Within a few weeks, Jade's nagging injuries subsided. These improvements in her physical and mental performance were a positive sign that Jade was able to prevent further decline and avoid the overtraining syndrome.

85. Are there any special nutritional considerations for youth athletes?

Physical activity and sports are important for children to participate in to help maintain physical and mental health, learn discipline and teamwork, and build confidence. Moderate physical activity and athletics provide many benefits for young athletes, including increased cardiovascular function, positive alterations in body composition (weight control), and development of a strong skeletal system. Nutritionally, youth athletes differ from adult athletes in that they must meet their required energy demands for physical activity as well as maintaining steady growth and maturation.

The youth athlete's physical growth (height and weight) is tracked yearly by his or her pediatrician. Proper growth is lineal and progressive with age. Growth or lack of growth can provide important insights into the youth athlete's nutritional status. Growth spurts and menstruation (females) occur in the adolescent years. Youth athletes who go through a growth spurt while participating in sports that emphasize weight classifications or restriction may risk delaying their normal growth and/or menarche.

Some youth athletes are pushed to achieve high levels of performance in competition. Higher level athletes often exercise numerous hours at a time placing significant

Moderate physical activity and athletics provide many benefits for young athletes, including increased cardiovascular function, positive alterations in body composition (weight control), and development of a strong skeletal system.

amounts of stress on their body, which can result in delayed menarche (females), slow growth and development, and possibly decreased bone density during low calorie intakes. Those athletes who have a chronically low energy (calorie) intake are more prone to the following conditions: late puberty, short stature, delayed menstruation or menstrual irregularities, poor bone health, increased incidence of injuries, elevated risk of developing disordered eating or eating disorders (see Question 74), and nutrient deficiencies.

Youth athletes who are eating well-balanced meals and snacks, three meals plus two to three snacks per day, should receive adequate amounts of vitamins and minerals (see **Table 30** for healthy snack options).

Youths who are not taking in enough energy (calories) may lack certain vitamins and minerals needed to maintain health. Calcium and iron (see Questions 51 and 52) are two important nutrients that are required for maturation; they should be supplemented if the healthcare provider finds a deficiency.

Table 30   Healthy Snack Options for Young Athletes

Pudding cups
Yogurt
Smoothies
Cheese cubes
String cheese
Milk/chocolate milk
Soy milk
100% fruit juices
Dried cherries, peaches, apricots, apples
Raisins
Peanut butter and whole-grain crackers
Graham crackers
Whole grain cereal or granola bars
Dry cereals
Fig bars

A key difference between youth and adult athletes is how the thermoregulatory system operates under exercising and extreme environmental conditions (see Questions 80 and 81). Youths have a less efficient thermoregulatory system (the thermoregulatory center is located in the **hypothalamus** of the brain and is responsible for temperature regulation), meaning that they are less tolerant to heat than adults. Youth athletes have a higher sweat threshold than adult athletes, which causes them to sweat much later during exercise. It is estimated that in similar hot environments a youth athlete will sweat about 400 to 500 milliliters per hour, whereas an adult will sweat 700 to 800 milliliters per hour. Youth athletes perspire less and produce more body heat for the same workload compared with adults. Their smaller body surface area results in less sweat forming and evaporating from the skin's surface, which in turn compromises cooling. A youth athlete's hypothalamus is not as fully developed as an adult's. This difference in hypothalamus development makes it harder for the young athlete's brain to detect and eliminate heat as efficiently as an adult, resulting in greater susceptibility to heat stress; therefore, young athletes must be encouraged to drink frequently during exercise to prevent dehydration and possible heat injury and must be monitored closely for any common signs of distress. Young athletes should also hydrate, take frequent breaks, wear appropriate clothing, and refrain from exercising during the hottest part of the day (see Question 81).

Similar to adult athletes, youth athletes feel the pressure to perform. Consequently, the use of ergogenic aids is tempting to many young athletes as a short cut to success. The indiscriminate use of supplements should be highly discouraged because of potential and

Hypothalamus
Region of the brain that contains a control center or many of the body functions, such as temperature regulation, hunger, and balance.

Nutritional and Exercise Considerations for Special Populations possibly dangerous side effects. In fact, the American Academy of Pediatrics does not recommend any supplement use by children under 18 years of age (see Question 95). Young athletes should be monitored closely by physicians, coaches, and parents and educated about the potential dangers of taking any substance that may decrease their performance and health and negatively impact their growth and maturation.

86. Are there any special exercise considerations for youth athletes?

When it comes to exercise, youth athletes should be highly encouraged to participate in regular daily activity for a minimum of 60 minutes. Historically, schools have been the bastion for after-school sports, physical education, recess, and children commuting to and from school by walking or riding their bikes. With the advent of the 21st century, these trends have been changing rapidly. Physical education in schools is no longer a daily activity. Children are more sedentary during recess. Busing and car pooling are the norm, and after-school sports are recruiting the more athletic population. The reduction in exercise trends among today's children has resulted in an ever-increasing sedentariness at school and home. This inactivity has created many youth public health issues that include childhood obesity, diabetes, and heart disease precursors such as hypertension, hypercholesterolemia, and hyperglycemia.

Children should be encouraged to participate in regular physical activity by parents, teachers, and healthcare providers. Some of the more important benefits of regular exercise in children include the following:

1. Stress reduction
2. Positive self-image

3. Increased readiness to learn

4. Maintenance of healthy weight

5. Proper growth

6. Optimum bone growth and development

7. Reduction of susceptibility to certain diseases (heart disease, diabetes, stroke, and certain cancers)

8. Promotion of strong, healthy bones, joints, and muscles

9. Improved sleep

A common concern for many parents today is the overwhelming amount of misinformation regarding some of the dangers of children participating in organized sports, weight lifting, and structured cardiovascular exercise. Concerns include the incidence of acute and chronic musculoskeletal injuries, growth-plate injuries, interference with normal growth and development, and burnout from overtraining.

Parents can be comforted by the fact that regular exercise is a safe and reliable means of helping their children develop a lifetime habit of physical activity. Youths should be encouraged to participate in organized sports and activities so that they can experience the same physiological and psychological benefits to exercise as adults. Youth sports injuries can be mitigated through appropriate supervision and coaching, medical screening, and correct wearing and use of personal protective equipment (helmets, pads, and eye protection). Personnel supervising youth activities must be knowledgeable, experienced, and aware of the impact that certain environmental conditions, such as heat and humidity, can place on youth athletes.

For many years, strength training was considered to be detrimental to the developing growth plates of youth athletes. Recent research, however, demonstrates that the benefits of youth strength training far outweighs the potential risks. A major concern to youth strength training was the possibility for growth-plate damage at the joints. Because youth athletes have not achieved complete growth-plate (**epiphyseal plate**) closure, it was believed that the joint was susceptible to increased injury from the use of weight resistance. Growth-plate closure occurs after the youth athlete has completed his or her growth spurt. This popular belief has now been disproved, as it has been demonstrated clearly that the correct application of resistance, recovery, technique, and qualified supervision has been very effective in helping eliminate youth growth-plate injuries. Many of the strength-training injuries incurred by youth athletes are primarily the result of poor program design and supervision, inappropriate use of weight loads, and poor technique—not necessarily because of any inherent physical limitation of the youth. The benefits of strength training are numerous and include increased bone, ligament, and tendon strength, increased lean body mass and reduced body fat, greater protection from injury, increased athletic performance, and enhanced body image and confidence. To help eliminate strength-training injuries, the following should be considered:

1. All youth strength training should be supervised by qualified personnel only.

2. Youths should be encouraged to develop good technique first. After a technique has been mastered, the steady application of resistance can follow.

3. Youths should be directed to use body-weight exercises (dips, pullups, pushups, body-weight squats, etc.) before using free weights. This will help them

A major concern to youth strength training was the possibility for growth plate damage at the joints.

Epiphyseal plate

Growth plate at each end of a long bone found in children and adolescents.

develop excellent body control, balance, and coordination.

4. Youths should experiment using resistance bands or springs, as they provide variable resistance through the exercise range-of-motion. These variable resistance devices can be helpful in reducing the potential for injury as the resistance is gradually applied to the muscle and joint when they are stretched.

5. Youths should be encouraged to train for strength and strength endurance with the use of medicine balls. Medicine balls provide an excellent alternative to traditional strength training and can be a fun way to workout. Medicine balls vary in weight and size, have the capacity to bounce, and are colorful, durable, and easy to grip. Youth athletes can do medicine ball drills either on their own or with a partner and can train in a very limited amount of space indoors or outdoors.

6. Youth athletes should be discouraged from doing maximal lifts because of their higher injury potential. Young athletes wanting to compete with one another should avoid free weights and should use calisthenic-type exercises instead. The exercises should be based on time (30 to 60 seconds) and are more fun and safer to conduct.

7. Effective strength development can be accomplished with two to three strength sessions per week that cover all the major muscle groups of the body.

When it comes to formal cardiovascular training programs such as running, cycling, rowing, and swimming, youth athletes should be highly encouraged to participate; however, cardiovascular benefits can also be accomplished with informal activities that involve spontaneous play where youths have fun just moving.

1. Youth athletes should be encouraged to participate in regular physical activity lasting at least 60 minutes, incorporating the large muscle groups of the body on most days of the week.

2. Youth athletes should be encouraged to make physical activity fun and spontaneous as opposed to being too structured.

3. Parents should be encouraged to exercise with their children to establish a lifetime of participation.

4. Youth athletes should not be preoccupied with unnecessary structure, including the rigid training schedules, training inflexibility, the use of heart rate monitors, and physiological testing, as these may decrease the fun of healthy competition.

5. Youth athletes can achieve cardiovascular benefits by training (formal exercise) at a minimum of 3 days per week for 30 minutes.

6. Youth athletes should be encouraged to participate in team sports to promote social interaction, cooperation, healthy competition, and pleasure.

7. Youth athletes should not be expected to train with the same methods as adults, as this can lead to injury or burnout.

8. Youth athletes, like adults, need proper rest and nutrition to avoid overtraining.

Formal training programs for youths must not overtrain or injure the athlete by working him or her too hard and/or too frequently. Youth athletes must be carefully monitored to ensure that injury and overexertion are eliminated through professional coaching. Youth training programs should be individually designed by a qualified strength and conditioning specialist using scientific training principals to maximize safety and effectiveness.

87. Does a masters athlete have specific nutritional requirements or require any special considerations?

A masters athlete, according to the World Masters Athletic Organization, is defined as a female over 35 years old and a male over 40 years old. As Baby Boomers age, the number of older men and women participating in recreational and competitive sports will increase correspondingly. For mature individuals to continue to remain active and competitive, certain chronological changes need to be understood and addressed in order for the masters athlete to train and compete at the highest possible levels. Recent **epidemiological** research shows that active adults are generally healthier; have less medical visits, fewer hospital stays, and use fewer medications; and have less chronic disease than their more sedentary counterparts. These older athletes will require a modified approach to their nutrition and training compared with younger athletes. Some of the key changes that occur as a result of aging involve differences in the athlete's energy needs, hydration status, vitamin/mineral requirements, and exercise capacities.

As the body matures, energy (carbohydrate, protein, fat), fluid, vitamin, and mineral requirements change. The nutritional needs for the masters athlete should focus on the specific effects of the aging process and his or her particular needs for training and competition. With advancing age, sedentary and nonathletic individuals will experience various physical and physiological alterations. Typical changes can include loss of lean body mass (muscle), diminished sensitivity to taste and smell, altered thirst reflex, reduced bone density, declining cardiovascular capacity, weakened immune system, and gastric deterioration.

Epidemiological

Information gathered from epidemiology, which studies how often disease occurs in certain groups and why. Results are then used to help treat and prevent disease.

The nutritional needs for the masters athlete should focus on the specific effects of the aging process and his or her particular needs for training and competition.

The masters athlete will need to consume a diet that is well balanced, offers variety, and is consumed in moderation to help maximize his or her fuel and recovery requirements. **Table 31** provides an overview of energy recommendations for the masters athlete.

The masters athlete should pay particular attention to his or her hydration needs. As individuals age, there is

Table 31 Energy Recommendations for Masters Athletes

Nutritional Requirements	Adjustments with Age
Total calories	• Total calorie (energy) intake usually decreases with age. • Masters athletes require more calories than sedentary adults.
Carbohydrates	• Carbohydrates are necessary to provide energy, fiber, vitamins, and minerals. • They help immune function by reducing stress hormones. • They should be 50% to 60% of daily intake: minimum of 5 grams per kilogram of body weight. • Older athletes store lower amounts of glycogen per unit of muscle mass and expend glycogen at faster rates compared with younger similarly trained athletes.
Proteins	• They are necessary to offset protein losses caused by continual breakdown (**catabolism**). • Needs are slightly higher to maintain a positive energy balance: 1.2 to 1.7grams per kilogram of body weight. • Protein intake that is too high can increase calcium loss, damage kidney function, and lead to **atherogenesis.**
Fats	• Fats are an essential source of fatty acids, fat-soluble vitamin absorption (A, D, E, and K), and energy source during moderate- to low-intensity exercise. • Needs remain at 25% to 30% of daily intake.

Catabolism

A process that breaks down larger molecules into smaller molecules (i.e., proteins to amino acids).

Atherogenesis

A build-up of plaque on the major arterial walls that reduces the diameter of the blood vessels causing decreased blood flow.

an inevitable reduction in total body water (intracellular and extracellular) resulting from a diminished thirst reflex, decreased kidney function, and irreversible changes in sweat gland sensitivity.

The American College of Sports Medicine (2007) established the fluid intake guidelines in **Table 32** for both older and younger athletes.

Table 32   American College of Sports Medicine's Fluid Intake Guidelines for Older and Younger Athletes

Before practice/competition: Drink 16 ounces (2 cups)
During practice/competition: Drink 20 to 40 ounces (2.5 to 5 cups) per hour with 5 to 10 ounces (0.5 to 1.25 cups) every 15 to 20 minutes.
After practice/competition: Drink 24 ounces (3 cups) of fluid for every pound lost. The extra 8 ounces (1 cup) accounts for additional urine and respiratory losses.

Masters athletes will also have an altered **Dietary Reference Intakes** for certain vitamins and minerals as a result of altered gastrointestinal efficiency. Most have higher needs for the vitamins C, E, B_6, B_{12}, riboflavin, and folate and for the minerals calcium, zinc, and magnesium. Masters athletes may have a decreased Dietary Reference Intakes for iron. Masters athletes who are taking medications for certain chronic and acute disorders will need to consult with their healthcare provider about the potential side effects that these drugs may have on exercise outcomes. For example, individuals with high cholesterol that are taking statin drugs may experience increased muscle soreness and decreased strength as a side effect.

Dietary Reference Intakes

A newer way to quantify nutrient needs and excesses for healthy individuals. The Dietary Reference Intakes expands on the older Recommended Dietary Allowances (RDA) and takes into consideration other dietary quantities such as Estimated Average Requirement, Adequate Intake, and Tolerable Upper Intake Level.

■ *Case Study*

Gloria, a 60-year-old avid walker, presents to her doctor with gastrointestinal upset and unexplained weight loss. Gloria is retired, and she exercises 60 to 90 minutes a day 5 to 7 days per week; she walks 45 to 60 minutes 5 to 7 days per week and strength trains two to three times per week for 20 to 30 minutes.

Gloria has noticed a few physical changes over the previous month: (1) She is feeling more soreness after strength training sessions; (2) she has lost 5 pounds in the last month without trying, and (3) she has been experiencing stomach pain and nausea after consuming some dairy products. Gloria's doctor refers her to a sports dietitian to help her evaluate and modify her current dietary intake.

During her appointment, Gloria states that the past month she has been very busy and realizes that the stomach pain and nausea after consuming milk products has diminished her overall appetite. Although her appetite has decreased, she has not changed her exercise program. From her food and exercise log, it is apparent that Gloria had not been consuming enough calories to support her exercise program and her body's recovery process, leading to fatigue and unintentional weight loss. Although with advancing age total energy (calorie) needs decrease, athletic adults must keep their energy intake high in order to perform, recover, and keep body weight stable. The stomach pains that Gloria has been experiencing are likely related to lactose intolerance. Gloria has been able to tolerate dairy products her entire life and is concerned by the sudden change. The dietitian details the mechanism of this change to Gloria and explains that the gastric acids in her stomach are changing along with the ability of her stomach to produce the enzyme lactase (which breaks down lactose). The declining enzyme lactase is the most likely cause of Gloria's stomach pains. Gloria is concerned that she will not be able to take in enough calcium to meet her needs (1,200 milligrams per day) if she is unable to tolerate milk products. The dietitian offers Gloria several options: (1) start consuming lactose-free dairy products, (2) take over-the-counter lactaid pills before consuming dairy products, (3) consume soy products that are fortified with calcium and vitamin D, and/or (4) consume a calcium supplement. The recommended calcium supplement for masters athletes is calcium citrate; this form of calcium is better absorbed in the acidic environment of the stomach and does not require additional stomach acid for absorption.

After one week of consuming lactose-free products and increasing overall calorie intake, Gloria reports that her workouts and recovery have improved. Her stomach pains have subsided, and she is no longer losing weight.

88. Do exercise requirements change for the masters athlete?

One of the more prominent physiological changes that occurs as a result of human aging is a decrease in aerobic capacity. It has been documented that oxygen consumption declines at a rate of 5 ml/kg/min per decade in athletes 25 years and older, which is approximately half that of inactive individuals (10 ml/kg/min per decade); therefore, inevitable declines in aerobic capacity with age can be slowed with an athlete who participates in a well-designed endurance training program at least three times per week.

Strength peaks at approximately 25 years of age and plateaus between 35 and 40 years of age. Individuals ranging in age between 40 and 65 can experience a loss of 25% in their peak muscular force. A masters athlete engaged in a well-designed strength training program should be able to maintain a significantly higher level of strength and performance compared with a sedentary adult. To reduce some unavoidable losses in overall strength throughout the years, the athlete should engage in resistance training at a minimum of two times per week.

Morphology

Change in form or shape.

As an athlete ages, **morphological** changes occur in the major joints of the body. Ligaments and tendons lose some of their elasticity and begin to stiffen with age; therefore, the older athlete must engage in a regular flexibility training program at least three times per week in order to maintain and/or improve flexibility. Before engaging in any type of flexibility program, the athlete should conduct a general warm-up that includes 5 to 10 minutes of light aerobic activity such as brisk walking or cycling. The warm-up is designed to decrease joint stiffness and increase joint range-of-motion by helping to increase the elasticity of the ligaments and tendons. This has the potential for reducing joint injury.

According to the Centers for Disease Control, the following exercise recommendations are made for persons 65 years of age or older. These recommendations are based on individuals who are generally fit and have no limiting health conditions according to their healthcare provider.

Older adults need at least the following:

Two hours and 30 minutes (150 minutes) of moderate-intensity aerobic activity (i.e., brisk walking) every week and muscle-strengthening activities on 2 or more days a week that work all major muscle groups (legs, hips, back, abdomen, chest, shoulders, and arms).

or

One hour and 15 minutes (75 minutes) of vigorous-intensity aerobic activity (i.e., jogging or running) every week and muscle-strengthening activities on 2 or more days a week that work all major muscle groups (legs, hips, back, abdomen, chest, shoulders, and arms).

or

An equivalent mix of moderate- and vigorous-intensity aerobic activity and muscle-strengthening activities on 2 or more days a week that work all major muscle groups (legs, hips, back, abdomen, chest, shoulders, and arms).

For greater health benefits, older adults should increase their activity to the following:

Five hours (300 minutes) each week of moderate-intensity aerobic activity and muscle-strengthening activities on 2 or more days a week that work all major muscle groups (legs, hips, back, abdomen, chest, shoulders, and arms).

or

Two hours and 30 minutes (150 minutes) each week of vigorous-intensity aerobic activity and muscle-strengthening activities on 2 or more days a week that work all major muscle groups (legs, hips, back, abdomen, chest, shoulders, and arms).

or

An equivalent mix of moderate- and vigorous-intensity aerobic activity and muscle-strengthening activities on 2 or more days a week that work all major muscle groups (legs, hips, back, abdomen, chest, shoulders, and arms).

89. Can traveling have an effect on my nutrition and performance?

Traveling can present several nutrition challenges for the athlete, including jet lag, food- or water-borne illness, and environmental stresses (altitude, temperature, cultural differences, and food availability). Today, more and more athletes are required to travel to compete, and thus, they must plan ahead in order to prepare themselves from making avoidable mistakes.

The mode and distance of travel can have a profound effect on the athlete's hydration status, food availability, sleep, mood, and proper gastrointestinal function. Short travel generally does not pose as many issues as long-distance travel. **Jet lag**, caused by traveling across time zones, can often lead to many of the issues stated previously here. Ideally, jet lag is best countered by adopting the time zone that competition will take place in a few days before arrival and then planning ahead to allow plenty of time before competition to adjust to the new environment. Research has shown that crossing three time zones requires one full day to recover. Each additional time zone above three requires an additional day; therefore, an athlete crossing six time zones would require four days to fully recover. A successful time zone shift will occur only if the athlete remains well hydrated, avoids alcohol and caffeine, and takes occasional naps during transit. Failure to comply with these simple rules can increase time zone adaptation to longer than the standard rule.

Today, more and more athletes are required to travel to compete, and thus, they must plan ahead in order to prepare themselves from making avoidable mistakes.

Jet lag

Fatigue felt when traveling between time zones that can affect mood, sleep, gastrointestinal function, and hydration status.

Airline travel can pose several obstacles for the athlete, but planning ahead can easily improve many of the following situations:

1. There is a limited availability of food and drink. Most airlines have stopped providing food on short flights or have limited food choices available for purchase. Drinks are provided, but usually only a 4-ounce serving or less. This can be remedied by bringing extra foods and drinks to ensure regular snacking and proper hydration.

2. Respiratory losses are enhanced by the dry cabin air. Fluid intake must be increased in order to offset these losses and to remain well hydrated. With limited availability of drinks, it is necessary that athletes bring beverages with them onboard.

3. Alcohol effects (see Question 63) increase when consumed onboard; therefore, alcoholic beverages should be avoided.

4. Caffeine generally poses no diuretic effect for those who are habitual consumers, but limiting consumption to 2 cups or less is recommended.

5. Gastrointestinal issues, such as constipation, are common when traveling. Consuming food high in dietary fiber with plenty of fluids often lessens the effects.

6. Keep blood circulating by regular walking, standing, and stretching; also, inquire about seats that provide extra leg room.

7. Wear comfortable clothing and footwear to ensure relaxation during travel.

Traveling by ground transportation (car, bus, or van) often poses less obstacles than airplane travel, but nevertheless, many of the same hurdles exist. Planning ahead by bringing the proper foods and beverages in addition to making frequent stops to stretch ensure better outcomes.

Preparing for the competing environment is crucial. Athletes must familiarize themselves with the conditions before leaving home to make certain that they have planned appropriately. Environmental factors to take into consideration include temperature, humidity, altitude, cultural differences, dietary customs (food choices, timing of meals), and meal preparation.

Temperature, humidity, and altitude should be assessed prior to arrival. In some cases, it is possible to become acclimated before travel so that the changes do not have a drastic effect on physical and mental performance. The cultural differences, dietary customs, and food preparation are important for the athlete to recognize when traveling both domestically and internationally. Some athletes may benefit from bringing a supply of foods and fluids that they enjoy to places where they might not care for food choices and/or the preparation of the food (**Table 33**).

Illness can often be a complication for athletes when traveling. Mild to severe vomiting, nausea, and diarrhea are unfortunately common. Sometimes these symptoms will subside over time, but severe cases should be addressed by a healthcare provider to assess whether medicine is warranted. The BRAT diet is often used to treat symptoms of diarrhea. BRAT is an acronym for bananas, rice, applesauce, and toast; these foods are bland, low in fiber, and tend to calm the symptoms of diarrhea.

Table 33   Perishable and Nonperishable Foods and Fluids for Traveling

Perishable—Keep Cold/Serve Cold	Nonperishable—Do Not Need Refrigeration
Sports drinks	Graham crackers
Bottled water	Vanilla wafers
Low-fat milk	Low-fat whole grain crackers
Yogurt	Animal crackers
Low-fat cheese sticks	Gingersnaps
Deli meats	Granola bars
Hard-boiled eggs	Cereal bars
Bagels	Sports bars
Fruit	Fig or fruit bars
Juices/juice boxes	Pretzels
	Bread sticks
	Canned fruit
	Canned puddings
	Dried fruit
	Dried cereals
	Peanut butter
	Canned tuna, chicken, or salmon

To avoid illness, water in certain countries should be avoided; this includes not consuming the tap water and ice or using tap water to brush teeth. Other foods to be cautious of include shellfish, unpasteurized milk products, unpeeled fruits and vegetables, and raw fish and other meats. Before consuming any foods, remember to check that all foods are cooked well.

Dining out is an important part of the traveling experience. It is not always viable to find hotel or housing accommodations with kitchens; thus, being restaurant and menu savvy can make certain that the athlete makes wise food choices. When eating out, choose foods that are broiled, boiled, baked, grilled, or steamed. Avoid foods that are fried or refried or in butter/cream/cheese sauce or gravy. At many restaurants, patrons can request that meals be prepared certain ways, and athletes should be encouraged to inquire if they do not see a pre-competition meal that they can tolerate. **Table 34** provides a list of healthy food choices when dining out.

Table 34   Healthful Food Choices When Dining Out

Carbohydrate Choices	Protein Choices	Lower Fat Options	Buffet-Style Eating
Low-fat or skim milk	Hamburger	Baked, broiled, roasted, boiled, poached, char-broiled items	Fill one plate first with vegetables, fruit, salads, whole-grain breads
Juice	Cheeseburger	Soft flour tortillas or corn tortillas	Broiled, grilled, or steamed meats, fish, chicken
Hot cocoa	Roast beef	Low-fat condiments, salad dressings	Avoid fried foods
Low-fat chocolate milk	Chicken breast	Vinaigrette dressings	Avoid cheesy, creamed foods
Whole-grain breads/rolls	Turkey	Steamed instead of fried rice	Baked potato instead of fries
Fruit muffins	Eggs	Salsa, picante sauce instead of sour cream and guacamole	Limit creamy salads, buttery croutons, and extra cheese on salads
Pancakes	Chili	Tomato or vegetable juice appetizer	Put garbanzo, kidney beans on salads
Toast	Meat sauce on pasta	Breads/rolls instead of chips as appetizers	Frozen yogurt or soft-serve ice cream for dessert
Bagels	Fish		Eat until you are full and then stop
Cornbread	Tuna or chicken salad		Avoid the "get your money's worth" mentality
Soups, including broth based, split pea, bean, minestrone, vegetable	Black, pinto, kidney beans		
Thick-crust vegetable pizza	Lentils		
Salads with corn, beets, carrots, three-bean salad	Tofu, bean curd stir-fry		
Pastas with marinara sauce	Lentil, bean, pea soup		
Pudding	Low-fat cottage cheese		

Before traveling, the athlete should be encouraged to research his or her destination in order to avoid the aforementioned pitfalls. An athlete who takes the time to do his or her homework should be well prepared for competition. Athletes must realize that months of hard work and preparation can be erased in a matter of hours if not nutritionally prepared for travel.

90. What do athletes need to understand about vegetarian diets?

Athletes can follow a vegetarian diet and still excel in sports. As a matter-of-fact, many professional athletes follow or have followed a vegetarian diet at some point in their athletic career, including Ricky Williams, Salim Stoudamire, Hank Aaron, Billie Jean King, Carl Lewis, and Edwin Moses. A vegetarian diet can be healthy as long as athletes are well versed in the diet, ensuring that they receive the proper nutrients. There are several types of vegetarian diets ranging from semi-vegetarian to vegan (**Table 35**).

Athletes can follow a vegetarian diet and still excel in sports.

Table 35   Types of Vegetarian Diets

Type	Animal Foods Included	Foods Excluded
Semi-vegetarian	Dairy products, eggs, poultry, fish	Red meats (beef, pork)
Pesco-vegetarian	Dairy products, eggs, fish	Beef, pork, poultry
Lacto-ovo-vegetarian	Dairy products, eggs	Beef, pork, poultry, fish
Lacto-vegetarian	Dairy products	Beef, pork, poultry, fish, eggs
Ovo-vegetarian	Eggs	Beef, pork, poultry, fish, dairy products
Vegan	None	All animal products and animal derivatives

Nutritional and Exercise Considerations for Special Populations

199

Often, athletes who choose to follow a vegetarian diet exclude animal products but fail to replace them with plant products that contain equal nutrients. These inadequate substitutions can lead to nutrient deficiencies; vegetarian athletes are most at risk for protein, iron, zinc, calcium, vitamin D, and vitamin B_{12} deficiencies (**Table 36**).

It has been proven that vegetarian diets can be nutritionally adequate as long as the athlete is knowledgeable about his or her body's requirements. Athletes who are vegetarians or are considering a vegetarian diet should consult with a registered dietitian if they have any questions or concerns. This will ensure that the athlete is on the right track to achieving his or her peak performance.

91. How does pregnancy change my nutrient and exercise needs?

Nutrient needs increase for women during pregnancy (see **Table 37**). Pregnant women on average require an extra 300 calories per day, but this can be more or less depending on individual needs. Some women may require additional calories, as they are more active, whereas others require fewer as they are less active. In May 2009, the Institute of Medicine provided new guidelines for weight gain during pregnancy (see **Table 38**) using prepregnancy BMI (see Question 68) to assess weight gain.

An exercise program offers many benefits for pregnant women, but the frequency and duration of exercise should be discussed with a physician before beginning

Table 36   Nutrient Considerations for Vegetarian Athletes

Nutrient	Function	Signs of Deficiency	Sources	Considerations
Protein	*Required for growth and repair of muscle and other body tissues *Large role in the formation of hormones, hemoglobin (blood), enzymes, and antibodies	*This is usually uncommon as there are so many vegetarian protein-rich foods	Beans, nuts, nut butters, soy, dairy, eggs, pork, poultry, fish	*Protein needs increase to 1.3 to 1.8 grams per kilogram of body weight (rather than 1.2 to 1.7 grams per kilogram in non-vegetarian athletes)
Iron	*Enzyme action for energy production *Hemoglobin synthesis and function *Collagen and elastin production	*Anemia; fatigue, poor performance	Beans, seeds, nuts, fortified grains and cereals, black-strap molasses, soy nuts, dried fruits, dark green vegetables, poultry, fish	*Recommended consumption of 1.8 times that of non-vegetarian athletes because of the lower bioavailability of iron in plant products (non-heme) versus animal products (heme) *Consume iron with vitamin C to help increase absorption
Zinc	*Eyesight *Immunity and wound healing	*Decreased immune function *Diarrhea *Poor appetite *Low thyroid hormone synthesis	Whole grains, fortified cereals, beans, nuts, seeds, dairy products, fish	*Recommend 50% more than non-vegetarians because of low bioavailability of zinc in plant sources

(Continued)

Table 36   Nutrient Considerations for Vegetarian Athletes (*Continued*)

Nutrient	Function	Signs of Deficiency	Sources	Considerations
Calcium	*Needed for strong bones and teeth *Muscle contraction *Blood clotting *Energy production *Keep immune system strong	*Osteoporosis	Milk and other dairy products, green leafy vegetables, broccoli, beans, tofu, salmon, sardines, calcium-fortified soy milk/soy food, calcium-fortified breads, cereals, and juices	None
Vitamin D	*Prevents cell damage *Antioxidant *Protects vitamins A and C and fatty acids	*Osteoporosis	Sunlight, green and leafy vegetables, wheat germ, whole grain products, fortified cereals, nuts, egg yolks	None
Vitamin B$_{12}$	*Helps build genetic material *Maintain nervous system *Development of red blood cells	*Weakness *Depression *Decreased sensation of the nervous system	Only found in animal foods: eggs, milk, milk products, fish, oysters, shellfish, fortified breakfast cereals, fortified soy milk	*Vegans will most likely be affected because B$_{12}$ is found in animal products only, but fortified foods and supplements can prevent deficiency

Table 37 Nutrient Needs for Pregnant Women

Nutrient	Function	Nonpregnant Recommendations	Pregnant Recommendations	Sources
Protein	*Required for growth and repair of muscle and other body tissues *Large role in the formation of hormones, hemoglobin (blood), enzymes, and antibodies	46 g/day	71 g/day	Beans, nuts, nut butters, soy, dairy, eggs, pork, poultry, fish, meat
Folate	*Promotes red blood cell production *Prevents birth defects of the brain and spine *Aids in protein metabolism *Lowers homocysteine levels therefore reducing risk of coronary artery disease	400 µg/day	600 µg/day	Whole grains, fortified cereals and grains, legumes, citrus fruits, green leafy vegetables, meats, fish, liver, kidney
Vitamin C	*Collagen formation *Wound healing *Immune function *Maintenance of blood vessels, bones, and teeth	14–18 years: 75 mg/day 19–50 years: 75 mg/day	14–18 years: 80 mg/day 19–50 years: 85 mg/day	Potatoes, broccoli, citrus fruits, melon, strawberries, tomatoes, green peppers, dark green vegetables, fortified juices

(continued)

Table 37   Nutrient Needs for Pregnant Women (*Continued*)

Nutrient	Function	Nonpregnant Recommendations	Pregnant Recommendations	Sources
Vitamin A	*Forms and keeps healthy skin and mucous membranes to increase resistance to infections *Necessary for night vision and tooth and bone development	14–18 years: 700 RAE μg/day 19–50 years: 700 RAE μg/day	14–18 years: 750 RAE μg/day 19–50 years: 770 RAE μg/day	Vitamin A fortified milk and dairy products, whole milk, cheese, egg yolk, liver, carrots, leafy green vegetables, sweet potatoes, pumpkins, winter squash, cantaloupe, apricots
Magne-sium	*Essential for biological processes *Activate enzymes involved in protein synthesis *Muscle contraction	14–18 years: 360 mg/day 19–30 years: 310 mg/day 31–70 years: 320 mg/day	14–18 years: 400 mg/day 19–30 years: 350 mg/day 31–70 years: 360 mg/day	Fish, nuts, beans, whole grains, green leafy vegetables, soybeans, wheat germ
Iron	*Enzyme action for energy production *Hemoglobin synthesis and function *Collagen and elastin production	18 mg/day	27 mg/day	Beans, nuts, seeds, meats, fortified grains and cereals, blackstrap molasses, soy nuts, dried fruits, dark green vegetables, poultry, fish

Table 38   Guidelines for Weight Gain During Pregnancy

Category	Weight Gain
Underweight (BMI < 18.5)	28–40 pounds
Normal weight (BMI 18.5–24.9)	25–35 pounds
Overweight (BMI 25–29.9)	15–25 pounds
Obese (BMI ≥ 30)	11–20 pounds

a program. The benefits of exercise during pregnancy include the following:

1. Reduced swelling of the hands and feet
2. Prevention of excessive weight gain
3. Alleviate insomnia and fatigue
4. Decreased incidence of leg cramps and varicose veins
5. Maintenance of bowel regularity
6. Improved circulation and posture
7. Reduction of backaches/back pain
8. Relief of pelvic and rectal pressure
9. Emotional wellness

Females must listen to their bodies during pregnancy. The pregnant female athlete must be aware that her body will be going through numerous physiological and hormonal changes that will impact her body's response to exercise. The female athlete should pay careful attention to these changes and make adjustments to her exercise intensity and duration accordingly. Pregnant females that experience any of the following symptoms during exercise should stop exercising immediately and call their physician: contractions, vaginal bleeding, faintness, dizziness, shortness of breath, heart palpitations, amniotic fluid leakage, persistent nausea or vomiting, hip or back pain, trouble walking, swelling, and/or numbness.

The pregnant female athlete must be aware that her body will be going through numerous physiological and hormonal changes that will impact her body's response to exercise.

Quick Fact

Low-impact activities such as walking, swimming (or other water activities), and stretching are highly recommended as they place less stress on the body and the fetus.

All female athletes who remain active during pregnancy will need to modify their nutrition and exercise program to ensure that they are gaining the appropriate amount of weight to guarantee proper growth and development of the baby. During this time, it is important to be monitored closely by a physician to make adjustments as needed.

Medications and Supplements

Why has my exercising heart rate changed since being put on beta-blocker drugs? Other than age-adjusted heart rate, what methods can I use to gauge my exercise intensity?

What are ergogenic aids?

What are ergolytics?

More . . .

Athletes need to be well-educated consumers. There are no shortcuts to athletic success. Successful performance is accomplished through hard work, determination, genetics, and a scientific approach to nutrition and exercise. Part Nine provides athletes with a comprehensive look at most commonly asked questions regarding medications and supplements so that they are able to make healthy, safe, and effective choices.

92. Why has my exercising heart rate changed since being put on beta-blocker drugs? Other than age-adjusted heart rate, what methods can I use to gauge my exercise intensity?

Beta blockers (beta-adrenergic blocking agents) are used to treat a variety of conditions such as high blood pressure, **glaucoma**, and **migraine headaches**. Beta blockers are designed to decrease blood pressure in hypertensive individuals by blocking the effects of **epinephrine** (adrenaline), a hormone released from the adrenal glands that increases heart rate, blood pressure, and blood glucose.

Beta blockers decrease resting and exercise heart rate and heart contractility and help to dilate blood vessels to reduce vascular resistance and increase blood flow. Beta blockers have potential side effects that include the following:

- Dizziness
- Weakness
- Fatigue
- Cold hands

Athletes using beta blockers frequently comment on the effects the drug has on their exercising heart rate.

Glaucoma

Eye disease that damages the optic nerve.

Migraine headaches

Painful, throbbing headaches that last 4 to 72 hours and often include nausea, vomiting, and photo sensitivity.

Epinephrine

Catecholamine released from the adrenal medulla that prepares the body for fight-or-flight response.

The beta blockers decrease heart rate at rest and during exercise. Many athletes find it difficult to monitor their exercise intensity using the standard age-adjusted heart rate formulas and usually fall below the heart rate required for a particular training zone. In fact, an athlete may never be able to reach his or her recommended target heart rate. There are significant individual differences in the effects of beta blockers; as a result, not all athletes respond the same way.

The effects of beta blockers on exercise capacity can be revealed by an exercise stress test or VO_2 max test, which can determine the impact that varying workloads have on the heart. Data collected from these scientific tests can be used to steer an athlete's training program safely and effectively (see Question 27); however, these tests are not always convenient or inexpensive; therefore, alternative methods must be considered. Other approaches to helping athletes determine their exercise heart rate include the following:

1. Use the RPE scale (see Question 25). This method can help to eliminate the need for heart rate monitoring during exercise, simultaneously being a convenient, accurate, and reliable method for gauging exercise intensity. An athlete exercising at 70% of his or her age-adjusted heart rate would look at a 12 to 13 on the RPE scale.

2. Decrease exercising heart rate by the same amount as resting heart rate while on beta blockers (see **Table 39**). For example, an athlete's resting heart rate before using beta blockers may be 80 beats per minute; after taking beta blockers, it is reduced to 60 beats per minute. The 20 beat-per-minute reduction at rest can be applied to the exercising heart rate. For an athlete working out at 70% of his or her

Table 39 Resting and Excercising Heart Rates With and Without Beta Blockers

	Without Beta Blockers	With Beta Blockers
Resting heart rate	80 beats per minute	60 beats per minute
Exercising heart rate (70%)	160 beats per minute	140 beats per minute

Athletes on beta blockers have alternatives to determining heart rate changes during exercise such as stress or VO$_2$ max testing, the use of the RPE scale, and/or the simple reduction equation method.

age adjusted heart rate, for example, 160 beats per minute, he or she may need to reduce his or her heart rate to 140 beats per minute. Although this is not a scientific approach, it may have merit for many athletes. There is no doubt that beta blockers affect resting and exercising heart rate.

Athletes on beta blockers have alternatives to determining heart rate changes during exercise such as stress or VO$_2$ max testing, the use of the RPE scale, and/or the simple reduction equation method. Whatever method an athlete selects to determine heart rate intensity, he or she should be assured that gains in his or her fitness should not be any different from athletes who are not taking beta blockers.

93. What are ergogenic aids?

Ergogenic aid

A substance, such as a steroid, that is used by athletes with the expectation that it will provide a competitive edge.

An **ergogenic aid** is any method that is used by athletes with the expectation that it will provide a physical or mental competitive edge. These methods can be nutritional, psychological, physiological, biomechanical, or pharmacological and are further explained in **Table 40**. Athletes should be aware that certain ergogenics are not necessarily performance enhancing.

Table 40 Type of Ergogenic Aids

Type of Ergogenic Aid	Description	Examples
Nutritional	Any supplement, food product, or dietary manipulation that enhances work capacity or athletic performance	Carbohydrate loading, creatine phosphate, amino acid supplementation, vitamin supplementation, glucose polymer drinks, sports gels, carbohydrate-loading drinks, liquid meals
Physiological	Any practice or substance that enhances the functioning of the body's various systems (e.g., cardiovascular, muscular) and thus improves athletic performance	Bicarbonate buffering, any type of physical training (e.g., endurance, strength, plyometric), blood doping via transfusions, the practice of warming up
Psychological	Any practice or treatment that changes mental state and thereby enhances sport performance	Visualization, sessions with a sport psychologist, hypnosis, pep talks, relaxation techniques
Biomechanical	Any device, piece of equipment, or external product that can be used to improve athletic performance during practice or competition	Weight belts, knee wraps, oversize tennis rackets and golf clubs, clap skates, body suits (swimming/track), corked bats
Pharmacological	Any substance or compound classified as a drug or hormonal agent that is used to improve work output and/or sport performance	Hormones (e.g., growth hormone, erythropoietin, **anabolic** androgenic steroids), amphetamines, caffeine, beta blockers, ephedrine

Medications and Supplements

Anabolic

To build up (i.e., amino acids to proteins).

94. What are ergolytics?

Ergolytics are any substance that may lead to a decrease in work productivity or physical/mental performance. Some examples of ergolytics include alcohol, energy drinks, and low-carbohydrate diets.

■ *Case Study*

Shareef, an Air Force fighter pilot, reports to the flight surgeon with symptoms of extreme **lethargy** and diminished mental focus. Shareef is very concerned as his environment in the aircraft places him under high **G forces**. Nothing significant was revealed in Shareef's physical exam. The flight surgeon suspects that Shareef might be experiencing some nutritional issues and refers him to a sports dietitian. The sports dietitian requests that Shareef keep a 3-day food and fluid log for review during the appointment. At first glance of Shareef's food log, it is obvious that he is not eating enough carbohydrates in his diet (causing an ergolytic effect) to fuel his muscles during high G maneuvering. During high G maneuvering, Shareef is required to contract the lower-extremity muscles of his body maximally to prevent blood from flowing into his legs. The dangers of not preventing blood flowing into the lower extremities could result in Shareef losing consciousness in the aircraft. On further review, Shareef reveals that he was trying to lose weight for an upcoming half marathon. He read an article on the Internet that promoted a low-carbohydrate diet as an effective way to lose weight. The sports dietitian cautions Shareef about the use of such fad diets and recommends for him to increase his carbohydrate consumption level back to at least 50% to 60% of his daily caloric intake. A week later, Shareef returns for a follow-up appointment with increased energy levels throughout the day and is performing better in the aircraft. In addition, his training for the upcoming half marathon also improved.

95. What should I consider before taking a supplement?

Supplements are not regulated by the **Food and Drug Administration** (FDA); therefore, the ingredients in

---

Lethargy

A state of being tired, lazy, or sluggish.

G forces

Force of gravity.

Food and Drug Administration (FDA)

The governing body responsible for ensuring the safety of foods sold in the United States. This includes oversight of the proper labeling of foods.

many of these products are not tested for safety or effectiveness. In 1994, under the Dietary Supplement Health Education Act, the Federal Government deregulated the supplement industry, allowing supplement manufacturers to make claims regarding the effect of products on structure/function of the body as long as they do not claim to diagnose, mitigate, treat, or prevent a specific disease. With the changes in the law, the multibillion-dollar (over $17 billion annually) supplement industry expanded, resulting in some unscrupulous practices that involved labels not matching the product's ingredients in addition to false claims. Some supplements may have none of the ingredients listed on the label, whereas others have an excessive amount. Many of the supplement ingredients may not have been laboratory tested and could potentially be harmful or even life threatening when consumed.

Quick Fact

The American Academy of Pediatrics does not recommend that any supplements be used by children under 18 years of age.

Before taking a supplement, the following questions should be asked:

1. What claims are being made regarding the benefits of the supplement?
2. Is it regulated by the FDA?
3. Has there been any independent scientific research conducted on this product?
4. Does it contain more than 100% of the Recommended Dietary Intake?
5. Is it safe?
6. Is it effective?

7. Is it free of contaminants?

8. Are there any potential food–drug interactions?

9. Can I get the same effect from eating a healthy diet?

10. What is the cost?

11. How is the dosage determined for the individual?

12. Will it cause an athlete to test positive for a banned substance(s)?

As one can see, supplements pose many unanswered questions and must be taken with extreme caution.

96. What does the U.S. Pharmacopeia label on my supplement mean?

Standards published by the **United States Pharmacopeia** (USP) in 2003 provide a set of guidelines for the quality, purity, manufacturing practices, and ingredients in supplement products. The USP has been in existence since 1820 and is a not-for-profit organization that is dedicated to setting public standards for the quality of healthcare products. In 2003, the USP developed quality standards for **dietary supplements**. The USP-verified mark is used only on supplements that have been through the extensive verification process required by the USP (see **Figure 18**). Before granting the USP-verified mark

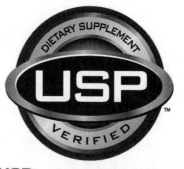

USP has tested and verified ingredients, product, and manufacturing process. USP sets official standards for dietary supplements. See www.usp-dsvp.org.

Figure 18   U.S. Pharmacopeia Verification Mark.

U.S. Pharmacopeia (USP)

A not-for-profit organization that establishes and verifies standards for the quality, purity, manufacturing practices, and ingredients in supplement products.

Dietary supplements

Products (other than tobacco) that are not intended to be used as a food or a sole item of a meal or diet. To be considered a dietary supplement, the product must contain one or more of the following dietary ingredients: vitamin, mineral, herb or other botanical, amino acid, dietary substance to supplement the diet by increasing total dietary intake or concentrate, metabolite, constituent, extract, or combination of any of these ingredients.

to a supplement, the USP will test the listed ingredients and verify the ingredients and amounts listed, test for contaminants, test that the supplement will break down and release ingredients in the body, and ensure that the product was manufactured using good manufacturing processes.

Manufacturers voluntarily choose to participate in the USP program to test and verify their dietary supplements. Athletes who purchase dietary supplements with the USP-verified symbol on the label may be getting a safer, higher quality product than those without the seal. Information on the products that have undergone the USP-verified process is available on the USP website.

Choosing a supplement manufactured by a well-known company may provide for a better product. The manufacturing and labeling used by larger, established companies will likely have better standards, such as an accurate listing of all the ingredients in the product and the dosage levels of all active ingredients.

Choosing a supplement manufactured by a well-known company may provide for a better product.

Some pharmaceutical manufacturers also make dietary supplements. The standards in place that these companies must use to have their drugs approved may also be used when they develop dietary supplements.

Although it is not guaranteed that supplement makers that also make pharmaceuticals will have better quality dietary supplements, it is one more thing athletes can look for when making supplement choices.

97. What is caffeine, and how can it affect my performance?

Caffeine is the single most widely used legal psychoactive substance in the world. Over 90% of Americans consume caffeine in some form every day. Caffeine is found in an array of beverages, foods, and pharmaceuticals that include coffee, tea, sodas, energy drinks, chocolate, aspirin, and even soaps and shampoos. The U.S. FDA lists caffeine as a "multiple purpose generally recognized as safe food substance." The primary source of caffeine used in the world is from the consumption of coffee. Caffeine content in coffee is dependent on the type of coffee consumed and how it is prepared. A single serving of coffee (6 ounces) can range between 40 to 120 milligrams of caffeine, with espresso having the least amount of caffeine and drip coffee having the most.

Caffeine is a bitter, white crystalline alkaloid that has very potent stimulating effects on the human central nervous system and metabolism. The stimulating effects of caffeine can temporarily ward off subjective feelings of drowsiness by improving alertness, focus, and reaction time, as well as providing a physical ergogenic benefit (see Question 93) to some athletes by decreasing the RPE during exercise (see Question 25). Caffeine is commonly consumed as a beverage but may also be consumed in higher concentrations in the form of pills or chewing gum.

The rate of entry of caffeine into the blood depends on how caffeine is ingested. Caffeine consumed as a beverage (coffee, tea, cola) enters the stomach quickly and is usually absorbed into the circulation and tissues within 45 minutes. Caffeine consumed in chewing gum bypasses the stomach and enters the bloodstream quicker than beverages through the membranes of the mouth, and the effects can be felt in as little as 10 minutes. Athletes requiring a quick energy boost before an event or practice may find using caffeine gum more efficacious than consuming beverages, but must be aware of the potential side effects if they are not accustomed to using this form of caffeine.

The half-life of caffeine, meaning the time required to metabolize half the amount of caffeine from the body, is generally accepted to be approximately 5 hours; however, the rate at which caffeine is metabolized by the liver can be influenced by many factors that include age, liver function, certain medications, pregnancy, and the levels of enzymes in the liver. Women taking contraceptives or who are pregnant may find that the half-life of caffeine doubles from 5 to 10 hours. Certain drugs such as Fluvoxamine (antidepressant) can increase the half-life to as much as 56 hours. Individuals suffering from serious liver disease have been shown to have a caffeine half-life as long as 96 hours. It is important for the athlete to understand how these factors influence caffeine metabolism; overconsumption of caffeine can have a paradoxical ergolytic effect (see Question 94) on the athlete if he or she is not careful.

Caffeine has been extensively researched over the years and has been proven to be a very effective ergogenic aid in the realm of athletics and sport. Studies have shown that caffeine can increase work capacity (endurance) from 7% to 51% in athletes. The variance in performance is dependent on the dose of caffeine consumed. Amounts of caffeine ranging between 3 to 9 milligrams per kilogram of body weight have been shown to be ergogenic (**Table 41**). Doses less or greater than the recommended ranges have not proven to be any more beneficial. In fact, some studies have shown there to be an ergolytic effect; therefore, it is imperative for an athlete who is looking to use caffeine as a potential ergogenic to discuss the protocol with a sports dietitian and experiment with varying dosages to establish the optimal amount for enhancing performance and reducing side effects.

Medications and Supplements

217

Table 41   Recommended Caffeine Consumption for Athletes

Amount	Time
3–9 milligrams per kilogram of body weight	60–90 minutes before exercise
1–3 milligrams per kilogram of body weight	Approximately every 2 hours during exercise

Despite caffeine's potential mental and physical ergogenic properties, the athlete needs to heed some precautions:

1. Caffeine consumed by novice users has the potential to produce a diuretic effect during initial use. The diuretic effect is usually transitory until the body develops a significant amount of tolerance. Recent research has demonstrated that consuming less than 300 mg of caffeine per day does not have a diuretic affect on novice or habitual caffeine consumers.

2. Using caffeine for the first time in hot environments has the potential to cause or exacerbate dehydration in the athlete, leading to possible thermal strain.

3. Overconsumption of caffeine above what is needed to produce an ergogenic effect can potentially lead to a condition referred to as **caffeinism**. Caffeinism is a dependency and can lead to reduced mental and physical performance (ergolytic effect).

4. Side effects associated with the overconsumption of caffeine commonly include nervousness, anxiety, irritability, muscle twitching, insomnia, and headaches. Tolerance to caffeine increases rapidly in regular users and requires higher dosages to produce the same effects as lower doses.

Caffeinism

A dependency on caffeine that can lead to reduced mental and physical performance.

5. Terminating caffeine use can also cause withdrawal. Withdrawal symptoms include headache, irritability, poor concentration, drowsiness, and stomach pains that usually occur within the first 12 to 24 hours and last up to 96 hours.

6. Overconsumption of caffeine during exercise may increase the chances of gastrointestinal upset (**hyperacidity**).

Hyperacidity

Increased hydrochloric acid secretion in the stomach, often causing a burning feeling in the stomach and esophagus.

Quick Fact

Recent research shows that caffeine use before competition or exercise may be related to an increased risk of muscle damage in some athletes, whereas in others, it may reduce post-workout muscle pain by 48% (more relevant to new exercisers). Caffeine users versus non-users have been shown to experience a lower rating of perceived exertion during both sprint and endurance exercise.

98. What are the pros and cons of using creatine for increasing performance?

Creatine supplementation use has been used extensively over the years by both professional and amateur athletes as an ergogenic aid (see Question 93). Creatine is produced naturally in the kidneys, liver, and pancreas of the body. Creatine is found in small amounts in foods such as red meat, pork, and fish.

In the human body, approximately two-thirds of all stored creatine is located in the muscle in the form of phosphocreatine, a high-energy phosphate molecule. The amount of creatine stored in the muscle is very limited—enough to last only a few seconds of high-intensity activity (sprinting). During high-intensity exercise, phosphocreatine is broken down very rapidly

Adenosine diphosphate

A high energy phosphate compound from which ATP is formed.

Adenosine triphosphate

A high energy phosphate compound from which the body derives its energy.

to donate a vital phosphate group to ADP (**adenosine diphosphate**) to remanufacture ATP (**adenosine triphosphate**), the basic unit of energy needed for muscular contraction (see the formula shown below). The capacity to maintain ATP levels with phosphocreatine is extremely limited and provides energy for approximately 10 to 15 seconds of intense exercise.

$$PCr \rightarrow Cr + P \rightarrow ADP + P \rightarrow ATP \text{ (energy)}$$

The mechanism behind using creatine as a supplement is to promote an increase in phosphocreatine levels within the muscle, similar to an endurance athlete using carbohydrate loading to increase glycogen levels in the muscle. By increasing the amount of phosphocreatine in the muscle, an athlete would be expected to increase the amount of ATP energy available during intense exercise. This in turn would translate into more power, faster recovery, a slower onset to fatigue, and ultimately better performance.

The use of creatine as a supplement has been accused of causing side effects in some of its users. Although clinical evidence is lacking in support of the side effects, athletes need to be aware that potential problems may exist. Some of the anecdotal reports of side effects include the following:

1. Cramping
2. Dehydration
3. Gastrointestinal distress (bloating, diarrhea)
4. Heat stress
5. Unintentional weight gain
6. Nausea

Creatine is a supplement and should be reviewed with a critical eye, as with all supplements that are manufactured without FDA regulation (see Question 95). Athletes run the same risks using creatine as any other supplement and need to do their homework before considering purchasing and using creatine. If an athlete has questions or concerns about using creatine as an ergogenic, he or she should consult with a licensed sports dietitian for advice and guidance.

Quick Fact

Not all creatine is created equal. Commercial creatine may not be as pure as creatine used in clinical laboratory testing. Impurities may result in side effects.

The following is a list of some of the pros and cons of using creatine. This information is an important resource for an athlete who is considering using creatine:

1. In order for creatine to be absorbed effectively, it should be taken with a simple carbohydrate source.

2. The use of creatine can lead to unintentional weight gain. The weight gain is probably caused by increased water retention in the cells. Coupled with a strength-training program, creatine can increase lean body mass.

3. The amount of phosphocreatine stored in muscle from creatine supplementation will depend on preexisting levels. The lower the initial amount, the greater will be the storage capacity and vice versa.

4. Some individuals are nonresponders (no effect), whereas others are high responders (strong effect) when supplementing with creatine.

5. Creatine is most effective during exercise of high intensity, lasting from 30 seconds to a couple of

Medications and Supplements

minutes. The supplement has been shown to be effective during repeated bouts of exercise such as multiple interval sprints.

6. Creatine supplementation appears to benefit athletes who are engaged in resistance training by increasing absolute strength levels (performing more repetitions with a faster recovery between sets).

7. Creatine does not appear to have a positive effect on endurance activities such as long-distance running or cycling; however, when it comes to short bursts of high-intensity activity during these events, such as sprinting at the end of a race, creatine has shown some benefit.

8. Creatine does not have to be front loaded (20 grams per day) for the first week to increase levels in the muscle. Creatine may be used in a smaller dose (5 grams per day) over a longer time period to load the muscles. This reduced dosage may help to minimize side effects in some athletes. Creatine levels increase approximately 20% in the muscles after supplementation.

9. Creatine may have a positive effect on endurance performance when used in conjunction with **Fartlek training**. More research is needed to quantify the possible benefits.

Creatine undoubtedly has potential ergogenic benefits for the strength and power athlete. Before using creatine, all athletes must consider the potential short- and long-term side effects of creatine on their health. Athletes using creatine in the hope of improving performance also run the risk of seeing little to no improvement in their performance, as laboratory studies showing a benefit may not translate into a field setting. One final thought for an athlete is the ethical

Fartlek training

A method of training the aerobic and anaerobic energy systems by regularly varying the intensity or speed during a workout session.

Athletes using creatine in the hope of improving performance also run the risk of seeing little to no improvement in their performance, as laboratory studies showing a benefit may not translate into a field setting.

consideration of an unfair advantage over athletes not using creatine.

99. Is flavored milk an effective post-workout recovery beverage?

Flavored milks, including chocolate, vanilla, strawberry, and coffee, are well liked and popular among children and adults. A significant amount of research has been conducted on the benefits of flavored milks, concluding that these beverages are nutritionally sound and are generally consumed more frequently than unflavored milk (see **Table 42**). Although higher in sugar than plain milk, flavored milks are only about 60 calories more than regular milk. This caloric difference is negligible when comparing the health benefits and nutrient content of flavored milks to sodas, juices, and sports drinks. The key points from the research on flavored milks are as follows:

1. Flavored milks are as nutritious as unflavored milks.
2. The calorie difference between flavored and unflavored milks is 60 calories (higher in flavored milks).
3. The amount of caffeine in some flavored milks (such as chocolate) does not cause hyperactivity in most children.
4. Calcium is absorbed equally in both flavored and unflavored milks.
5. Flavored milk intake does not spoil the appetite or displace other healthy foods.
6. Flavored milks can be part of a healthy, well-balanced diet.

The benefits of chocolate milk as a recovery beverage are unequivocal. Research conducted in 2006 on endurance cyclists who consumed a post-exercise recovery drink

Table 42   Milk's Unique Nutrient Package

Benefits for Bones and Beyond

Milk contains nine essential nutrients, making it one of the most nutrient-rich beverages you can enjoy. Drinking 8 ounces of delicious and nutritious milk can help you get one step closer to meeting the Dietary Guidelines for Americans' recommended three servings of low-fat or fat-free milk or milk products a day. Just one 8-ounce serving of milk is an excellent source of calcium, vitamin D, protein, and other key nutrients. Read on to learn just how important milk's nutrients are for good health.

Calcium 30% Daily Value

An 8-ounce serving of milk provides 30% of the Daily Value of calcium. Calcium helps build and maintain strong bones and teeth. This mineral also plays an important role in nerve function, muscle contraction, and blood clotting.

Vitamin D 25% Daily Value

When fortified, a glass of milk provides about 25% of the Daily Value for vitamin D. Vitamin D helps to promote the absorption of calcium and enhances bone mineralization. Milk is one of the few dietary sources of this important nutrient.

Protein 16% Daily Value

The protein in milk is high quality, which means that it contains all of the essential amino acids or "building blocks" of protein. Protein builds and repairs muscle tissues. An 8-ounce glass of milk provides about 16% of the Daily Value for protein.

Potassium 11% Daily Value

Potassium regulates the body's fluid balance and helps to maintain normal blood pressure. It's also needed for muscle contraction. By providing 11% of the Daily Value of potassium, milk contains more than the leading sports drink.

Vitamin A 10% Daily Value

A glass of milk provides 10% of the Daily Value of vitamin A. This nutrient helps maintain normal vision and skin. It also helps to regulate cell growth and maintains the integrity of the immune system.

Vitamin B$_{12}$ 22% Daily Value

Vitamin B$_{12}$ helps to build red blood cells that carry oxygen from the lungs to the working muscles. Just one 8-ounce glass of milk provides about 22% of the Daily Value for this vitamin.

Riboflavin 26% Daily Value

Milk is an excellent source of riboflavin, providing 26% of the Daily Value. Riboflavin, also known as vitamin B$_2$, helps convert food into energy—a process crucial for exercising muscles.

Niacin (Niacin Equivalents) 10% Daily Value

Niacin is important for the normal function of many enzymes in the body and is involved in the metabolism of sugar and fatty acids. A glass of milk contains 10% of the Daily Value for niacin.

Phosphorus 25% Daily Value

Phosphorus helps strengthen bones and generates energy in your body's cells. Providing 25% of the Daily Value, milk is an excellent source of phosphorus.

Source: National Dairy Council

showed that chocolate milk, with its high carbohydrate and moderate protein content, was an effective alternative for recovery from exhausting, energy-depleting exercise.

In 2009, a study conducted on collegiate soccer players concluded that post-exercise consumption of chocolate milk was found to provide possibly superior muscle recovery when compared with a high-carbohydrate recovery beverage with the same amount of calories. Although there were no differences between the effects of the beverages on performance tests, subjective ratings of soreness, mental fatigue, physical fatigue, or other measures of muscle strength, the chocolate milk drinkers had significantly lower levels of creatine kinase in their circulation after exercise. Creatine kinase is a marker of muscle tissue damage. The higher the levels of creatine kinase in the circulation, the greater the muscle tissue damage, and vice versa. Overall, milk has been proven to be an effective recovery beverage for athletes of all ages and levels. Milks benefits go beyond recovery, as milk also helps to rehydrate athletes and provide essential nutrients needed after strenuous exercise.

Quick Fact

Many athletes are now favoring flavored milk as their post-exercise recovery drink instead of sports drinks. Its unique combination of ingredients provides greater benefits than sports drinks alone.

Clearly, milk and milk products provide many low-cost health and recovery benefits. How can athletes include more into their diets? The following provides some suggestions:

1. Drink more low-fat and non-fat unflavored and flavored milks in place of sodas, juices, and sports drinks.

2. Add milk to coffee and tea.

3. Consume yogurt with meals and snacks.

4. Blend and enjoy milk-based fruit smoothies.

5. Include moderate amounts of low-fat cheeses into meals and snacks.

6. Enjoy ice cream and frozen yogurt in moderation.

7. Instead of adding milk to your coffee, add coffee to your milk.

PART TEN

More Information

Where can I find more information about sports nutrition and exercise?

100. Where can I find more information about sports nutrition and exercise?

A plethora of information is available on nutrition and exercise, but not all the information is accurate or reliable. As an athlete, make sure that the information you obtain comes from a qualified and reputable source.

According to the American Dietetic Association, a registered dietitian is a healthcare professional who has an extensive scientific background in food, nutrition, biochemistry, and physiology.

According to the American Dietetic Association, a registered dietitian is a **healthcare professional** who has an extensive scientific background in food, nutrition, biochemistry, and physiology. His or her knowledge is applied to promoting health, preventing disease, and providing counseling and education. A registered dietitian must complete (1) at least a 4-year degree at an American Dietetic Association accredited college program, (2) a supervised practice program or internship, (3) a national examination from the Credentialing Board of Dietetic Registration, and (4) mandatory continuing professional education. A board certified sports dietitian continues his or her education to specialize in the following areas of nutrition: (1) sports nutrition, (2) cardiovascular health, (3) weight management and wellness, and (4) prevention and treatment of disordered eating and eating disorders.

Healthcare professional

A person who is medically educated to provide advice.

Exercise physiologist

A healthcare provider (not a personal trainer) with an academic degree in exercise physiology from an accredited college or university.

According to the American Society of Exercise Physiologists, an **exercise physiologist** is a healthcare provider who has an academic degree in exercise physiology from an accredited college or university. Exercise physiologists are able to identify the physiological mechanisms that underlie physical activity; the comprehensive delivery of treatment services concerned with the analysis, improvement, and maintenance of health and fitness; rehabilitation of heart disease and other chronic diseases and/or disabilities; and the professional guidance and counsel of athletes and others interested in athletics, sports training, and human adaptability to acute and chronic exercise.

The following websites provide a wealth of reputable nutrition and exercise information. Many of the websites contain downloadable handouts and book references as well.

Nutrition

Sports, Cardiovascular, and Wellness Nutrition: http://www.scandpg.org/

American Dietetic Association: http://www.eatright.org

Gatorade Sports Science Institute: http://www.gssiweb.com/

Australian Institute of Sport: http://www.ausport.gov.au/ais/

National Dairy Council: http://www.nationaldairycouncil.org/NationalDairyCouncil/

The Vegetarian Resource Group: http://www.vrg.org/

Exercise

National Strength and Conditioning Association: http://www.nsca-lift.org/

American College of Sports Medicine: http://www.acsm.org/

American Academy of Pediatrics: http://www.aap.org/

American Society of Exercise Physiologists: http://www.asep.org/

Quest Sports Science Center: http://www.questssc.com

Disordered Eating

National Eating Disorders: http://nationaleating
disorders.org/

Something Fishy: http://www.something-fishy.org/

Female Athlete Triad: http://www.femaleathletetriad.
org/

Young Women's Health: http://www.youngwomens
health.org/

Academy for Eating Disorders: http://www.
aedweb. org/

MEDA: http://www.medainc.org/

Supplements

National Library of Medicine database: http://www.
ncbi.nlm.nih.gov/PubMed

Consumer Lab: http://www.consumerlab.com

Natural Medicine Comprehensive Database: http://www.
naturaldatabase.com

Dietary Supplement Information Bureau: http://www.
supplementinfo.org

US Anti-Doping Agency: http://www.usanti
doping.org/

World Anti-Doping Agency: http://www.wada-ama.
org/en/

Masters Athletes

CDC Guidelines for Older Adults: http://www.cdc.
gov/physicalactivity/everyone/guidelines/olderadults.
html

World Masters Athletics: http://www.world-masters-
athletics.org/

Coaches

Institute for Sports Coaching: http://www.institute forsportcoaching.org/

Credential Check

It is always important to check credentials in order to ensure that you receive accurate scientific information that will improve, not hurt, your health and perform-ance. Here is a list of credentials and their meanings to help you start your search on the right foot. Remember that the best approach to optimal performance is the multidisciplinary approach. Athletes should not rely on one provider to give them all of the answers. It is important to seek out the appropriate professional to answer specific sports-related questions. Avoid using your primary-care provider to answer all of your sports exercise- and nutrition-related questions, as these can be better answered by an exercise physiologist or a sports dietitian.

RD = Registered Dietitian

CSSD = Board Certified Specialist in Sports Dietetics

LD = Licensed Dietitian

MS = Master of Science

PhD = Doctor of Philosophy

CSCS = Certified Strength and Conditioning Specialist

ATC = Certified Athletic Trainer

CPT = ACSM/NSCA Certified Personal Trainer [SM]

HFS = ACSM Health Fitness Specialist

CES = ACSM Certified Clinical Exercise Specialist®

RCEP = ACSM Registered Clinical Exercise Physiol-ogist®

CIFT = ACSM/NCPAD Certified Inclusive Fitness Trainer

BIBLIOGRAPHY

American College of Sports Medicine. (2007). Position stand on the female athlete triad. *Medicine and Science in Sports and Exercise, 39*, 1867–1882.

Baechle, T. R., & Earle, R. W. (2000). *Essentials of Strength Training and Conditioning* (2nd ed.). Champaign, IL: Human Kinetics.

Borg, G. A. V. (1982). Psychophysical bases of perceived exertion. *Medicine and Science in Sports and Exercise, 14*, 377–381.

Burke, L., & Deakin, V. (2006). *Clinical Sports Nutrition* (3rd ed.). New York: McGraw-Hill.

Dunford, M. (2006). *Sports Nutrition: A Practice Manual for Professionals* (4th ed.). USA: American Dietetic Association.

Fink, H. H., Burgoon, L. A., & Mikesky, A. E. (2009). *Practical Application in Sports Nutrition* (2nd ed.). Boston: Jones and Bartlett Publishers.

Fragakis, A. S. (2003). *The Health Professionals Guide to Popular Dietary Supplements* (2nd ed.). USA: American Dietetic Association.

Gilson, S. F., Saunders, M. J., Moran, C. W., Corriere, D. F., Moore, R. W., Womack, C. J., & Todd, M. K. (2009). Effects of chocolate milk consumption on markers of muscle recovery during intensified soccer training. *Medicine and Science in Sports and Exercise, 41*, S577.

Karp, J. R., Johnston, J. D., Tecklenburg, S., Mickleborough, T. D., Fly, A. D., & Stager, J. M. (2006). Chocolate milk as a post-exercise recovery aid. *International Journal of Sport Nutrition and Exercise Metabolism, 16*, 78–91.

Levine, B. D., & Stray-Gunderson, J. (1997). "Living high-training low": Effect of moderate-altitude acclimatization with low-altitude training on performance. *Journal of Applied Physiology, 83*, 102–112.

Position of the American Dietetic Association. (2006). Nutrition intervention in the treatment of anorexia nervosa, bulimia nervosa, and other eating disorders. *Journal of the American Dietetic Association, 106*, 2073–2082.

Position of the American Dietetic Association and Dietitians of Canada. (2003). Vegetarian diets. *Journal of the American Dietetic Association, 103*, 748–765.

Position of the American Dietetic Association, Dietitians of Canada, and the American College of Sports Medicine. (2009). Nutrition and athletic performance. *Journal of the American Dietetic Association, 109*, 509–527.

Sawka, M. N., Burke, L., Eichner, R., Maughan, R. J., Montain, S. J., & Stachenfeld, N. S. (2007). Exercise and fluid replacement. American College of Sports Medicine position stand. *Medicine and Science in Sports and Exercise, 39,* 377–390.

Wilmore, J. H., & Costill, D. L. (2004). *Physiology of Sport and Exercise* (3rd ed.). Champaign, IL: Human Kinetics.

Glossary

Acclimatization: A process in which the body undergoes physiological adjustments or adaptations to changes in environmental conditions such as altitude, temperature, and humidity. The physiological changes enable the body to function better in the new climate.

Acid reflux: An abnormal condition in which the valve between the stomach and the esophagus is not functioning properly; therefore, the acid from the stomach rises into the esophagus, causing a burning feeling.

Active stretch: When an athlete applies the force for the stretch.

Adenosine diphosphate: A high-energy phosphate compound from which ATP is formed.

Adenosine triphosphate: A high-energy phosphate compound from which the body derives its energy.

Adipose tissue: Made of adipocytes, which store excess dietary fat not used by the body.

Aerobic: In the presence of air or oxygen.

Ambient temperature: Air temperature.

Amenorrhea: The absence or abnormal cessation of menstruation; defined as less than four cycles per year.

Amino acids: The basic structural building units of proteins.

Anabolic: To build up (i.e., amino acids to proteins).

Anaerobic: In the absence of air or oxygen.

Anemia: A condition that occurs when less than the normal number of red blood cells are in the blood or when the red blood cells in the blood do not have enough hemoglobin.

Anorexia athletica: A subclinical condition in which individuals practice inappropriate eating behaviors and weight-control methods to prevent weight gain and/or fat increases. Anorexia athletica does not meet the criteria for a clinically defined eating disorder, but the behaviors exhibited are on a continuum that could lead to the more severe clinically recognized eating disorders.

Anorexia nervosa: A clinical condition manifested by extreme fear of becoming obese, a distorted body image, and avoidance of food. Anorexia nervosa can be life threatening and requires medical and psychiatric treatments.

Antibodies: Part of the immune system that helps to combat and neutralize foreign bodies such as viruses, bacteria, and parasites.

Anticatabolic substance: A nutritional compound that slows the breakdown process in the body (catabolism), thus tilting the metabolic balance toward increased tissue building (anabolism).

Atherogenesis: A build-up of plaque on the major arterial walls that reduces the diameter of the blood vessels causing decreased blood flow.

Atmospheric pressure: Force per unit area exerted against a surface by the weight of air above that surface. One atmosphere equals 14.7 pounds per square inch.

Ballistic stretching: Often called the bounce technique; the movement is rapid with no hold at the end of the stretch.

Basal metabolic rate (BMR): The minimum amount of energy required to sustain life in the waking state. The basal metabolic rate is usually measured in the laboratory under very rigorous conditions.

Binge eating disorder: Falls under the category of eating disorder not otherwise specified. It is characterized by recurrent episodes of binge eating, a lack of self-control during binge eating, and marked distress after a binge.

Bioavailable: The amount of an ingested nutrient that is absorbed and available to the body.

Bioelectrical impedance analysis: A body composition assessment technique that measures the resistance to flow of an insensible electric current through the body; the percentage of body fat is then calculated from these impedance measurements.

Blood glucose: Amount of glucose circulating in the bloodstream.

Blood glucose response: Measurement of how circulating blood glucose responds to an increase or a decrease in food intake.

Blood lipid profile: A blood test that determines the amount of fat in the form of cholesterol and triglyceride in the circulation.

Blood sodium concentration: Concentration of the amount of sodium in the blood. Normal levels are between 136 and 145 mmol/L.

Blood volume: Volume of blood circulating in a person's body. The blood consists of red blood cells and plasma.

Body mass index (BMI): An indicator of nutritional status that is derived from height and weight measurements. Body mass index has also been used to provide a rough estimate of body composition even though the index does not account for the weight contributions from fat and muscle.

Body surface area: Calculation or measurement of the body's surface.

Bonking: A condition in which an athlete experiences extreme fatigue and an inability to maintain the current level of activity. It is also known as "hitting the wall" and results when the body has depleted muscle and liver glycogen levels.

Borg scale: Is also known as the Rating of Perceived Exertion scale. The scale has a numerical value attached to it, increasing by 1 unit starting at 6 and ending at 20. A rating of 6 (no exertion at all) would be given by someone relaxing, whereas a rating of 20 (maximal exertion) could be given by an athlete at the end of a hard sprint. The scale is an effective tool in helping athletes to select an exercise intensity without having to use a heart rate monitor.

Bulimia nervosa: A clinical condition characterized by repeated and uncontrolled bingeing in which a large number of calories are consumed in a short period of time, followed by purging methods such as forced vomiting or use of laxatives or diuretics.

Caffeinism: A dependency on caffeine that can lead to reduced mental and physical performance.

Carbohydrate loading: A method of increasing the cell's glycogen content beyond its usual capacity.

Carbohydrates: The main source of energy for all body functions, particularly brain and muscle functions; necessary for the metabolism of other nutrients.

Cardiac drift: An increase in heart rate as a result of decreased central blood volume caused by dehydration or blood loss.

Cardiac output: The volume of blood being pumped by the heart in 1 minute: cardiac output = stroke volume × heart rate.

Cardiorespiratory: Function of both the heart and lungs.

Cardiovascular strain: Strain put on the cardiovascular system (heart and blood vessels).

Caseinated protein: Long peptide-bonded structure that is digested at a slower rate than whey protein. Caseinated protein is found in milk.

Catabolism: A process that breaks down larger molecules into smaller molecules (i.e., proteins to amino acids).

Cellular glycogen: Amount of glycogen stored in the cells.

Cellular level: The smallest structure that is capable of independent functioning in an organism.

Central nervous system: Body system that consists of the brain and spinal cord.

Circumference method: A method that uses height, weight, and various body locations that are then compared with a standard table. Women are measured at the neck, waist, and hip, and men are measured at the neck and waist.

Colon: Part of the digestive system whose main function is to extract salt, water, and certain vitamins before they are eliminated from the body.

Combustion: A process that produces heat.

Compartment syndrome: Increased pressure caused by inflammation within a muscle compartment of the body, impairing its blood supply.

Complex carbohydrates: A carbohydrate composed of two or more linked simple-sugar molecules.

Core temperature: Temperature in the body's core, 98.6°F.

Coronary artery disease: Progressive narrowing of the coronary arteries.

Cramps: Painful involuntary muscle contractions that usually occur in the body's lower-extremity muscles (calves, hamstrings, quadriceps).

Decalcification: A loss of calcium from teeth and bones.

Dehydration: A condition resulting from a negative water balance (i.e., water loss exceeds water intake).

Delayed onset muscle soreness: A phenomenon of muscle pain or muscle stiffness that generally occurs 12 to 48 hours after exercise.

Diastole: A resting phase of the heart where blood refills the chambers of the heart.

Dietary fiber: A complex carbohydrate obtained from plant sources. It is not digestible by humans. Although dietary fiber provides no energy for cellular activity, it does help maintain a healthy digestive system, lower blood cholesterol levels, and regulate blood glucose levels.

Dietary Reference Intakes: A newer way to quantify nutrients needs and excesses for healthy individuals. The Dietary Reference Intakes expands on the older Recommended Dietary Allowances (RDA) and takes into consideration other dietary quantities such as Estimated Average Requirement, Adequate Intake, and Tolerable Upper Intake Level.

Dietary supplements: Products (other than tobacco) that are not intended to be used as a food or a sole item of a meal or diet. To be considered a dietary supplement, the product must contain one or more of the following dietary ingredients: vitamin, mineral, herb or other botanical, amino acid, dietary substance to supplement the diet by increasing total dietary intake or concentrate, metabolite, constituent, extract, or combination of any of these ingredients.

Disordered eating: Observed when athletes alter their eating patterns, in an unsafe way, in an attempt to lose weight or maintain weight at a lower than normal weight.

Diuretic: A drug or other substance that tends to promote the formation and excretion of urine.

Dual-energy X-ray absorptiometry: A method of body composition assessment that involves scanning the body using radiography technology to distinguish between fat and lean body tissue.

Duration: The amount of time an athlete spends exercising.

Dynamic stretching: A method of stretching using sports-specific movements to increase flexibility.

Eating disorder not otherwise specified: An eating disorder that does not meet all of the criteria needed for it to be diagnosed as either bulimia nervosa or anorexia nervosa but that meets the criteria to be labeled as a true eating disorder.

Eccentric: Movements that cause the muscle to contract while lengthening. Examples of eccentric muscle actions include going down stairs, downhill running, and the lowering of weights in the gym.

Electrolytes: Potassium, chloride, and sodium are found in sweat. They are needed to maintain normal metabolism and function. For example, sodium is essential in maintaining fluid balance.

Energy drinks: Drinks that advertise that they will improve physical and mental performance. Many add caffeine, vitamins, and herbal supplements that often act as stimulants.

Enzymes: Proteins that accelerate chemical reactions.

Epidemiological: Information gathered from epidemiology, which studies how often disease occurs in certain groups and why. Results are then used to help treat and prevent disease.

Epinephrine: Catecholamine released from the adrenal medulla that prepares the body for fight-or-flight response.

Epiphyseal plate: Growth plate at each end of a long bone found in children and adolescents.

Ergogenic aid: A substance, such as a steroid, that is used by athletes with the expectation that it will provide a competitive edge.

Ergolytic: Any substance that may lead to a decrease in work productivity or physical/mental performance.

Essential body fat: Fats found within the body that are essential to the normal structure and function of the body.

Eumenorrhea: A term used to describe normal menstruation consisting of at least 10 menstrual cycles per year.

Exercise-induced rhabdomyolysis: A condition resulting from an acute skeletal muscle injury that causes the muscle cell membrane to break open, spilling its contents into the circulation.

Exercise physiologist: A healthcare provider (not a personal trainer) with an academic degree in exercise physiology from an accredited college or university.

Fad diets: Weight-loss programs or supplements that promise to deliver quick weight loss with minimal effort.

Fad exercise: Exercise programs or ideas that promise to deliver quick gains with minimal or maximal effort.

Fartlek training: A method of training the aerobic and anaerobic energy systems by regularly varying the intensity or speed during a workout session.

Fat: A wide group of compounds that may be either solid or liquid at room temperature.

Fat-free mass: The weight of all body substances except fat. Fat-free mass is primarily made of organ weight and the skeletal muscles, including minerals, protein, and water.

Fat mass: The portion of body composition that is fat. Fat mass includes both fat stored in the fat cells and essential body fat.

Fat-soluble vitamins: A group of vitamins that do not dissolve easily in water and require dietary fat for intestinal absorption and transport into the bloodstream. The fat-soluble vitamins are A, D, E, and K.

Fatigue: Physical or mental exhaustion from overexertion.

Female athlete triad: A group of three interrelated conditions, typically diagnosed in young female athletes—disordered eating, menstrual irregularities, and osteopenia/osteoporosis.

Fibrosis: A condition in which fibrous connective tissue replaces muscle fibers.

Flexibility: The range of motion about a joint.

Food allergy: Occurs when the immune system attacks a food protein and produces an adverse reaction such as itching, hives, rash, swelling, labored breathing, and/or loss of consciousness.

Food and Drug Administration (FDA): The governing body responsible for ensuring the safety of foods sold in the United States. This includes oversight of the proper labeling of foods.

Food intolerance: Irritation of the digestive system when a food is unable to be broken down.

Free radicals: Highly reactive molecules, usually containing oxygen, that have unpaired electrons in their outer shell. Because of their highly reactive nature, free radicals have been implicated as culprits in diseases ranging from cancer to cardiovascular disease.

Frequency: The number of training sessions per week.

Fructose: A simple sugar, commonly found in fruits, that is known for its sweet taste.

G forces: Force of gravity.

Galactose: A simple sugar found in milk.

Gastric emptying: The rate at which foods and fluids exit the stomach.

Gastrointestinal distress: Distress that occurs in the upper or lower gastrointestinal tract that can negatively impact sports performance.

Glaucoma: Eye disease that damages the optic nerve.

Gluconeogenesis: The formation of glycogen from fatty acids and proteins rather than from carbohydrates.

Glucose: One of the most commonly occurring simple sugars in nature. Humans rely on glucose for cellular energy.

Glycemic index: An index for classifying carbohydrate foods based on how quickly they are digested and absorbed into the bloodstream. The more quickly blood glucose rises after ingestion, the higher the glycemic index.

Glycogen: The major carbohydrate stored in animal cells, mainly in the muscle cells and some in the liver. Glycogen is converted to glucose and released into circulation, as needed, by the body.

Glycogen synthesis: A biological process for increasing the amount of glycogen in the liver and muscle cells.

Glycolysis: Breakdown of glucose into energy.

H2 blockers: Anti-hypertensive medications that is used to control blood pressure.

Healthcare professional: A person who is medically educated to provide advice.

Heart rate monitor: A wireless device that consists of a transmitter (strapped around the chest) and a watch-like receiver (worn around the wrist).

Heme iron: A well-absorbed form of iron found in red meats, fish, and poultry.

Hemoglobin: A complex protein–iron compound in the blood that carries oxygen to the cells from the lungs and carbon dioxide away from the cells to the lungs.

Hormone: A complex chemical substance produced in one part or organ of the body that initiates or regulates the activity of an organ or group of cells in another part.

Hunger: An unpleasant sensation that an individual experiences when circulating blood glucose decreases; it can be alleviated through eating.

Hydrostatic weighing (underwater weighing): The gold standard of body composition determination that involves weighing a person while he or she is totally immersed in water.

Hyperacidity: Increased hydrochloric acid secretion in the stomach, often causing a burning feeling in the stomach and esophagus.

Hypobaric: An environment, such as at high altitude, that involves low atmospheric pressure.

Hyponatremia: A lower than normal concentration of sodium in the blood, caused by inadequate excretion of water or by excessive water in the circulating bloodstream.

Hypothalamus: Region of the brain that contains a control center or many of the body functions, such as temperature regulation, hunger, and balance.

Immune system: A system within an organism that protects against disease.

Inactive rest: An extended period of inactivity.

In-season: Part of the training schedule that consists of a high amount of activity and competition.

Insulin: A naturally occurring hormone secreted by the cells of the pancreas in response to increased levels of glucose in the blood. The hormone acts to regulate the metabolism of glucose, fats, and proteins.

Intensity: How hard an athlete works during training and competition.

Involuntary dehydration: When an athlete does not have control over his or her fluid consumption or the rate at which the fluids can be lost and absorbed.

Isometric: Muscular contraction resulting in no change in the muscle's length.

Jet lag: Fatigue felt when traveling between time zones that can affect mood, sleep, gastrointestinal function, and hydration status.

Lactase: A digestive enzyme that breaks lactose into the simple sugars glucose and galactose.

Lactate: The biproduct of cellular glucose breakdown.

Lactate threshold testing: Considered, by sports scientists, to be one of the single most important markers of success in endurance-related activities.

Lactic acidosis: A condition in which there is a significant accumulation of hydrogen ions in the blood and tissue, leading to muscle acidification.

Lactose: A sugar found in milk that is composed of glucose and galactose.

Lactose intolerance: The body's inability to digest significant amounts of lactose (sugar found in milk and other dairy products) because of low or absent levels of the enzyme lactase.

Lanugo: Fine, white hair that grows usually on the arms and chest of those who are severely underweight. The hair serves as a mechanism to keep the body warm where there is not enough body fat available to do so.

Lean body mass: The portion of a body's makeup that consists of fat-free mass plus the essential fats that comprise those tissues.

Lean proteins: Protein sources that are low in saturated or trans fats, including beans, nuts, nut butters, eggs, chicken, turkey, fish, and soy.

Lethargy: A state of being tired, lazy, or sluggish.

Low body fat: Body fat levels below 5% for males and 12% for females.

Major minerals: The minerals required by the body in amounts greater than 100 milligrams per day. The major minerals include calcium, phosphorus, magnesium, sodium, chloride, potassium, and sulfur.

Metabolite: A substance produced by the process of metabolism or vital for a certain metabolic process.

Metabolize: The breaking down of carbohydrates, proteins, and fats into smaller units; re-organizing those units as tissue building blocks or as energy sources; and eliminating waste products of the processes.

Micronutrient: Essential nutrients (i.e., vitamins and trace minerals) required in only small quantities (milligrams and micrograms) by the body.

Migraine headaches: Painful, throbbing headaches that last 4 to 72 hours and often include nausea, vomiting, and photo sensitivity.

Mitochondria: Powerhouses of the cell that burns carbohydrates, fats, and proteins for energy.

Monounsaturated fat: A type of fat that is shown to reduce the incidences of heart disease.

Morphology: Change in form or shape.

Muscle dysmorphia: A type of disordered body image in which individuals have an intense and excessive preoccupation and/or dissatisfaction with body size and muscularity. Muscle dysmorphia is most prevalent in male bodybuilders and weight lifters.

Myoglobin: Found mainly in muscle tissue; serves as a storage site for oxygen.

Nerve conduction: The transmission of impulses throughout the nerves in the body.

Night eating syndrome: A disordered eating pattern that is characterized by 50% or more of total caloric intake eaten after 7 p.m., sleep disturbances, morning anorexia, and frequent eating during the night that lasts for over 3 months. Night eating syndrome is usually associated with overweight or obese individuals.

Non-essential body fat: Fat found in adipose tissue. Non-essential body fat is also called "storage fat."

Nonheme iron: A less well-absorbed form of iron found in fruits, vegetables, grains, and nuts.

Non-rapid eye movement (NREM): The first stage of sleep where very little dreaming occurs. The purpose behind non-rapid eye movement sleep is to help the body physically repair itself from the previous day's activities.

Off-season: Part of the training schedule that consists of less than the normal amount of activity.

Oligomenorrhea: A condition in which the female menstrual period is irregular, with cycles occurring only four to six times per year.

Osteoporosis: Means "porous bone" and usually affects older adults. This disease is characterized by decreased bone mineralization and is a product of poor bone formation during puberty. This disease weakens the bones and results in an increased susceptibility to fractures.

Overload: A method of training that requires the physiological systems of the body to be increasingly stressed to ensure continued improvement.

Overtraining syndrome: A condition that results in a steady decrease in physical and mental performance over time. Symptoms include constant tiredness, persistent muscle and joint soreness, inability to focus, and/or feeling burnt out or stale.

Oxidized: A chemical reaction with oxygen.

Palatability: Acceptable taste or flavor.

Pandemic: An epidemic of a disease that is spreading through human populations across a large region such as a continent or several continents (worldwide).

Passive stretch: Requires the use of a device or person to apply the force for the stretch.

Peptide-bonded protein: A molecular chain compound composed of two or more amino acids joined by peptide bonds.

Percent body fat: The amount of fat mass found on the body expressed as a percentage of total body weight.

Periodization: A method of training that varies the volume and intensity of training over a period of time to prevent overtraining.

Periodized program: A phased program that allows the body to adapt and recover in order to achieve optimal gains.

Plaque: A build-up of lipids (fats) in the arteries of the heart that reduces blood flow.

Plethysmography (BodPod): A technique that measures the volume of air displaced by an object or body. In body composition assessment, air displacement plethysmography is used to determine the volume of the body so that the density of the body can be determined.

Polyunsaturated fat: A type of unsaturated fat that has been shown to prevent heart disease.

Progression: A principle that requires an athlete's training program to be progressively advanced over time to ensure improvement (peaking) and reduce injury or burnout.

Proprioceptive neuromuscular facilitation: Often referred to as the stretch–hold–contract technique. This method of stretching usually requires a partner with a certain level of expertise to perform.

Protein: Made up of amino acids that act as the building blocks for muscles, blood, skin, hair, nails, and the internal organs.

Rapid eye movement (REM): This second stage of sleep involves a substantial amount of dreaming and is essential to helping individuals recover mentally. During the rapid eye movement cycle, the mind attempts to process and organize all of the information that it has encountered during the day.

Rating of perceived exertion (RPE): Often referred to as the Borg scale (see Borg scale).

Recommended Dietary Intake: The daily amount of nutrients needed to satisfy approximately 98% of healthy individuals.

Registered dietitian: An individual trained to provide food and nutrition information and who has successfully passed the national registration exam for registered dietitians.

Respiratory: Includes airways, lungs, and respiratory muscles that allow gas exchange.

Resting metabolic rate (RMR): The minimum amount of energy required to meet the energy demands of the body while at rest. The resting metabolic rate is typically measured instead of BMR because it is only slightly higher than BMR and is determined under less rigorous conditions.

Running economy test: A laboratory assessment to determine the efficiency of a runner's muscles, joints, and pulmonary system (lungs).

Satiety: Being full or satisfied.

Saturated fat: Fat that can cause an increase in cholesterol levels and that increases the risk for heart disease.

Simple carbohydrates: A form of carbohydrate that exists as a monosaccharide or disaccharide.

Situational awareness: Aware of the surrounding environment within space and time.

Skinfold calipers: An instrument that is used to measure the thickness of skin folds in millimeters.

Soy protein: A protein source made from soybeans.

Specificity: A training principle that necessitates an athlete to specifically train for the sport or activity.

Static stretching: Referred to as the stretch-hold technique. It begins by moving the joint and muscle through a range of motion until the stretch sensation is felt in the belly of the muscle.

Stitches: Similar to cramps. They occur in the upper body typically between the lower ribs and pelvis.

Stomach pangs: A sharp feeling of pain in the stomach.

Stress fracture: An overuse injury in which the fatigued muscle can no longer bear the stress and transfers it to the bone.

Sucrose: A commonly consumed sugar also known as table sugar. It is composed of glucose and fructose.

Supercompensate: A method that increases glycogen stores beyond the cell's normal capacity.

Sweat test: A method to determine sweat rate, electrolyte losses, and overall fluid needs.

Syncope: A sudden drop in blood pressure that causes dizziness and possible fainting.

Systole: The contraction phase of the heart that ejects blood into the circulatory system.

Tapering: A scheduled decrease in the volume and intensity of training six or more days prior to competition. The purpose is to allow for recovery from training and replenishment of glycogen stores in the liver and muscle.

Thermoregulation: The control of heat production and heat loss for maintaining normal body temperature.

Thirst reflex: A signal by the body to help regulate fluid balance.

Total daily energy expenditure: Total amount of calories (energy) expended by the body over a 24-hour period.

Total energy intake: Total amount of calories (energy) needed by the body over a 24-hour period.

Trace minerals: Minerals required by the body in quantities less than 100 milligrams per day. The trace minerals include iron, zinc, chromium, fluoride, copper, manganese, iodine, molybdenum, and selenium.

Training intensity: The amount of effort (low, moderate, high) required to perform a specific exercise.

Training volume: The total amount of work done during a training period.

Trans fat: Considered to be an unhealthy source of fat that often leads to cardiovascular disease if ingested in high amounts.

U.S. Pharmacopeia (USP): A not-for-profit organization that establishes and verifies standards for the quality, purity, manufacturing practices, and ingredients in supplement products.

Unsaturated fat: A heart-healthy fat that has the potential to lower cholesterol levels and reduce heart disease.

Urinary losses: Loss of macronutrients and micronutrients via urination.

Variation: Comes from changing workloads, exercises, or both.

Vascular: Blood vessels in the circulatory system.

Vascular resistance: The resistance to blood flow that must be overcome to push blood through the circulatory system.

Venous return: The transportation of blood from the cells through the veins back to the heart.

VO$_2$ max test: An accurate scientific laboratory method of measuring an athlete's cardiorespiratory (aerobic) capacity. The VO$_2$ max test determines the maximum amount of oxygen in milliliters that an athlete can consume per kilogram of body weight per minute during a graded exercise test.

Volume: The amount of work done during an exercise bout.

Voluntary dehydration: Normally occurs when an athlete ignores the need to drink, has a poor thirst reflex, and/or refuses to carry a water bottle and consume fluids before and during exercise.

Waist circumference: A measure of abdominal girth taken at the narrowest part of the waist as viewed from the front.

Waist-to-hip ratio: A comparison of waist girth to hip girth that gives an indication of fat deposition patterns in the body.

Water-soluble vitamins: A class of vitamins that dissolve in water and are easily transported in the blood. The water-soluble vitamins are the B vitamins, vitamin C, and choline.

Whey protein: A biproduct of cheese manufacturing. It is a short peptide-bonded protein and is rapidly digested and absorbed into the circulation (bloodstream). Whey protein is found in yogurt and cottage cheese (the liquid on the surface of the product before it is mixed).

Wingate power test: The gold standard to assess muscle power, muscle endurance, and muscle fatigability.

Work capacity: The capacity to do work.

Index

Index